Patient Teaching by Registered Nurses

Studies in Nursing Management, No. 9

Philip A. Kalisch, Series Editor

Professor of Nursing, Politics
and Economics of Nursing
The University of Michigan

Beatrice J. Kalisch, Series Editor

Titus Professor of Nursing and
Chairperson, Parent-Child Nursing
The University of Michigan

Other Titles in This Series

Patient Teaching by Registered Nurses

by
Ann Minnick

UMI RESEARCH PRESS
Ann Arbor, Michigan

Produced and distributed by
UMI Research Press
an imprint of
University Microfilms International
Ann Arbor, Michigan 48106

Library of Congress Cataloging in Publication Data

Minnick, Ann.
 Patient teaching by registered nurses.

 (Studies in nursing management ; no. 9)
 Revision of the author's thesis—Northwestern University,
1980.
 Bibliography: p.
 Includes index.
 1. Patient education. 2. Nurses—Attitudes. 3. Nurses—
Psychology. I. Title. II. Series. [DNLM: 1. Teaching—
Methods—Nursing texts. 2. Patient education—Methods—
Nursing texts. W1 ST929N no. 1 / WY 105 M665p]
 RT90.M56 1982   610.73   82-17623
 ISBN 0-8357-1378-4

Contents

List of Figures

List of Tables

Preface

The purpose of this book is to present research on patient teaching that may be useful in making decisions in nursing management and nursing education. The descriptions of the methodology used in this work may also be helpful in designing the always improving studies of the future.

One aspect of nursing which this study cannot appropriately reflect is the commitment of nurses to their patients and the profession. Staff nurses, the subjects of this study, were invariably amiable in taking on the added burden of a nurse-researcher despite the many other demands of their jobs. Their informal discussions on how nursing practice might be improved indicated that the profession has many members of which it can be proud. I would like to thank these nurses and the many other nurse executives and educators who encouraged me in the completion of this work.

This book is based on a study done during doctoral education made possible, in part, by an HEW National Research Service Award (5-F31-NU-05007-03). Many people contributed helpful advice so that the investigation could be completed. Robert J. Menges, Ed.D. was a supportive reviewer and teacher. Thomas D. Cook, Ph.D. and B. Claude Mathis, Ph.D. assisted in clarifying theoretical and statistical issues. Kathryn McCarville, R.N. patiently endured the inter-rater reliability testing procedures as well as the classification of all clinical data. Any errors which exist within the work are, of course, my own.

In the most direct sense, the book exists due to University Microfilms International Research Press. It is a pleasure to acknowledge their assistance as well as that of the series editors, Philip and Beatrice Kalisch.

On a personal level, the book's completion reflects the support of my family and friends. My husband, Cole, and my parents, James and Helen Fenley, have always been a source of encouragement. To them goes my sincere, continuing gratitude.

1

The Study Problem

Some of the leading causes of death in the United States adult population are cardiac and vascular diseases, cancer and diabetes. At the present time there are no simple cures or preventative vaccines available to combat these problems. To some extent, the degree of control of these illnesses appears to depend upon careful adherence to certain regimens of diet, activity and/or medication. As practitioners well know, complete adherence is unlikely. In an early study of 3,800 outpatients in Boston, only 42% of the fracture patients were found to be following the recommendations of their physicians and less than 60% of the diabetics were found to have taken medications and diets correctly (Berkowitz, 1963). In the last two decades, researchers have begun to examine the causes of such nonadherence, the results of such actions, and methods to increase what has come to be called compliance, i.e. "the extent to which the patient's behavior coincides with the clinical prescription" (Sackett and Haynes, p. 1, 1976).

In order to comply with a regimen, the patient must first understand the regimen's prescriptions. Many organizations including the U.S. National Center (U.S. National Center for Health Services Research and Development, 1973) and the Blue Cross (Blue Cross, 1974), have endorsed the idea that teaching patients is cost effective. In fact, some studies have shown knowledge on the part of the patient to be associated with increased compliance while others have failed to show such a relationship (Sackett and Haynes, 1976; Cohen, 1981). Failure to demonstrate a positive correlation between knowledge and compliance does not, however, negate the possible worth of patient education as an aid to adjustment to illness. It does not release the clinician from the ethical obligation of informing the patient about the illness and treatments.

In an American Hospital Association survey of 2,680 community, non-federal, general hospitals, 45.5% of the hospitals were able to cite specific line responsibility for the coordination of patient teaching. Where a line designation could be made, the department of nursing was cited as responsible in the majority of cases. In all cases, registered nurses were most frequently reported as being involved in the planning and teaching of inpatients (Lee and Garvey, 1978).

It thus appears that there is a need for patient education to be studied as it relates to compliance and that there is a need for nurses' teaching behavior to be studied as a variable in the educational efforts to improve compliance. These inquiries are necessary not only for the improvement of individual practice but for comprehensive nursing management decisions. Practitioners wish to know the impact of various types and styles of teaching on patient behavior. Nursing administrators wish to have information on which to base decisions regarding the structure, design and resources necessary for patient education within institutions.

A Pilot Study Leads to New Questions

A study was proposed to examine two variables (health beliefs and health locus of control) and their relationship to compliance, to patient education and to each other. The two variables, when studied separately, had resulted in varying ability to predict compliance. The variables also presented an opportunity to attempt detailed description, within a social psychological framework, of patient education provided by nurses as it relates to compliance.

Purpose of the Pilot Study

It was proposed that adult inpatients who had a diagnosis of diabetes mellitus and their nurses be asked to participate in the study. Consenting patients and nurses would be interviewed for demographic data and opinions on the health locus of control and the health belief scales before patient teaching began. The first teaching session would then be tape recorded and patients interviewed on the scales prior to discharge. After one month, the patients would be contacted via telephone regarding the scales and perceptions of their compliance with the suggested regimen. Physicians would be contacted via mail regarding their observations and perception of the patients' adherence.

The study was limited to patients who had been diagnosed as having adult onset diabetes but who were not currently hospitalized for treatment of diabetic complications involving the eye or extremities. The study was also limited to patients who were receiving diabetic instruction for the first time at that particular agency.

Care had been taken to secure an institution which had strong supportive policies for nurses, and well developed standards for diabetic teaching. The agency's nurses and clinical coordinators estimated that the five hundred bed community hospital would have four to eight patients per week who would meet the subject criteria.

Findings of the Pilot Study

From May 11 to June 8, 1979, fifty-five diabetics were identified via the Kardex as possible subjects. Table 1.1 describes this group. Despite the seemingly large number of potential subjects, only two patients were interviewed and no teaching tapes were made. The reasons for not including these patients in the study are presented in Table 1.2.

A surprisingly large number were inappropriate subjects because no future self-care of the diabetic condition was deemed possible either due to anticipated early death resulting from another condition or indefinite continued inability to care for self. Childhood onset of diabetes and diabetic complications of the eyes or extremities were reasons for the elimination of only a small number of subjects. The two subjects who were interviewed were not taped because the nurses labeled these patients as knowledgeable about diabetes. No further teaching was planned. The twenty-four patients who were assessed as incapable of self-care in the future were not taught. In three of these cases, families were going to assume care responsibilities and they were taught about diabetes.

The group of special interest are those patients described as "potentially teachable" (Table 1.3). By interviewing these patients' nurses, it was ascertained that only two cases (both new diabetics) received the complete teaching package as outlined by the agency's standard of care. Five cases appear to have received no teaching. The nurses gave different reasons for not teaching these patients including short hospitalizations, pressure on nurse due to short staffing and changes in patient assignment. The researcher, however, could find no significant difference in these factors between those patients who were assessed or assessed and received some teaching and those who were lost to teaching.

The "potentially teachable" patients who were assessed but not taught raise another interesting point. Assessment sheets provided by the hospital were used in two cases; assessment methods in the other cases cannot be verified. The two reasons given by the nurses for not teaching these patients were: (1) that the patient had been diabetic for a number of years and thus must know about it and (2) the patient had been in the hospital many times and was incorrigible in the matter of diabetic management. In the former case, it appears the nurses were associating duration of the condition with knowledge and compliance and in the latter case, it appears, the nurses judged further teaching to be an ineffective strategy.

Table 1.1.   Description of Potential Subjects
55 Diabetics, May–June, 1979

Factor	Number
Sex	
Male	33
Female	22
Age	
Range	25–92
Average Age	63
Admitting Diagnosis	
Cancer	15
Cerebral vascular disease	6
Heart disease	5
Diabetes	5
Amputation or vascular disorder of extremities	5
Asthma	3
Benign prostatic hypertrophy	3
Fracture of the femur	3
Pancreatitis	2
Biopsy of suspicious lesion	2
Fever of undetermined origin	1
Cataracts	1
Pleural effusion	1
Gastrointestinal bleeding	1
Gastrointestinal examination	1
Systemic lupus erythematosus	1

Table 1.2.   Status of Patients as Possible Subjects

Category	Number
Not eligible, no further self-care post-hospitalization	24
Not eligible, childhood onset type	5
Not eligible, diabetic complications	5
Not eligible, no confirmed diagnosis	1
Not eligible, psychiatric complications	2
Not eligible, no treatment ordered	2
Not eligible, discharged rapidly or nurse did no assessment	14
Eligible and interviewed	2

Table 1.3. Potentially Teachable Patients

Type of Teaching Done	Number of Patients
Complete teaching per hospital guidelines	2
Assessed by nurse but no teaching done	10
Assessed by nurse with some teaching done	11
No teaching due to short hospitalization and/or change in nursing staff patterns	5
Total	28

Why Is There So Little Teaching?

The agency had no figures with which to compare these survey findings. Supervisors and unit nurses voiced surprise over the number of ineligible patients. Two additional months of monitoring confirmed this pattern of admission although there was a slight increase in the number of "potentially teachable" diabetics admitted.

The results of this initial investigation lead to the conclusion that factors related to the nurse's decision to teach and the kind of teaching done should be probed further. In an institution with primary nursing, strong administrative support, developed standards of teaching and good physical resources, many of the common reasons given for failure to teach are not present yet teaching is not taking place as envisioned.

Need for the Study

The nursing literature also supports the need for further study. During the last fifteen years, there has been an abundance of materials and articles cited by the Nursing Index as being concerned with patient teaching. The majority of the articles have dealt with specific content to be taught to patients with discrete, diagnosed illnesses. The next most frequently appearing are reports on the incidence, types and outcomes of patient teaching. These studies most often describe a teaching approach or approaches and report or compare outcomes. Designs are usually of the quasi-experimental type.

Studies from the nursing literature on incidence and type of teaching have been few in recent years although administrative manpower studies, often privately funded by individual institutions, have documented some types of patient teaching. A landmark study was done by Pohl in 1965. In a questionnaire completed by 1500 members of the American Nurses' Association, Pohl found that the concept of patient teaching held by nurses was unclear at best. It is of significance that 37.2% of those refusing to answer the questionnaire indicated, when recontacted, that they gave direct nursing care but did not teach.

In more recent times, the 1977 National Survey of Registered Nurses found 61.1% of the registered nurses reporting that their practice included "instructing and counseling patients and families in areas of health promotion and maintenance including involving patients in planning their own care" (Moses and Roth, 1979). In the same study, 65.5% of the nurses reported "instructing patients in the management of defined illnesses." The report did not ask nurses to indicate specific actions or the level or depth of these activities. General duty nurses who had baccalaureate degrees were more likely to report patient and family teaching as a part of their routine than those general duty/staff nurses who held either the associate degree or diploma.

In her review of the patient teaching literature, Redman suggested lack of educational preparation might be related to inadequacies in patient teaching (Redman, 1976). Her review also cited studies which investigated other factors which might affect patient teaching. Among the factors identified were: (1) lack of clarity as to what patient teaching is, (2) preparation levels of registered nurses, (3) confusion about the nurse's role in teaching, (4) lack of expectation by employers and (5) the use of information as a controlling power. Few of these studies were multifactorial and randomized. Several of the studies were not of recent execution. The use of theoretical frameworks was often limited or nonexistent.

In a review of the non-research literature, Cohen reported many of the same barriers to patient education as those discussed by Redman (Cohen, 1981). The three principal factors cited were poor preparation to teach, the number of teachers covering the same content and the low priority often assigned by administrative and supervisory personnel. In considering the second factor, non-research articles often pointed out the difficulties associated with standardization of content, delegation of teaching responsibility and communication with large numbers of staff of diverse backgrounds.

It thus appears that there is a need for nursing studies of patient teaching that include the following points in their design:

1. Actual observation of teaching instead of reliance on self-report.
2. Randomization.
3. Reference to a theoretical framework.
4. A multifactorial approach.
5. An identification and differentiation of the different types of patient teaching.

Purpose and Theoretical Framework

The purpose of this study is to identify factors, within a theoretical framework, that may be related to the type and incidence of patient teaching done by registered nurses in the general hospital setting. This study begins to specify factors needed to assess the likelihood of patient teaching by registered nurses. This attempt to determine factors might result in future work on development of criteria to encourage patient teaching or to evaluate the efforts currently being made to support patient teaching by registered nurses.

A framework must be identified to avoid some of the problems associated with past work. As noted in the pilot study, locus of control has been a valuable concept in examining and predicting behavior. It is a part of Rotter's social psychological theory (Rotter, 1975). A special health locus of control scale has been developed (Wallston, et al., 1978). Another framework which has demonstrated its usefulness in the study of factors affecting behavior is Fishbein and Ajzen's behavior intentions theory. Its chief strength appears to be its examination of both personal attitudes and social pressures.

These two frameworks, which will be explored in the next chapter, seem to contain the five elements previously identified by Redman as possibly influencing patient teaching. Moreover, there is some basis (also explored in Chapter 2) for believing that the two frameworks may be related. Use of both these frameworks in a single study may result in more information regarding this relationship as well as increased direction with which to answer the central question of the study: What factors are related to the type and incidence of teaching done by registered or graduate nurses in a general hospital?

Research Questions

General Question: What factors are related to the types and incidence of patient teaching done by registered nurses in the general hospital?

Question I: What is the relationship between health locus of control and type and incidence of patient teaching by registered or graduate nurses in a general hospital?

Question II: What is the relationship between the variables of the behavior intentions model and the type and incidence of teaching done by registered or graduate nurses in a general hospital?

Question III: What is the relationship between the health locus of control concept and the behavior intentions model?

*Rationale for Question I: Relationship Between
Health Locus of Control and Patient Teaching*

Control was previously described as a possible factor in nurses' willingness to teach and in their actual teaching behaviors. The health locus of control scale examines one aspect of control, i.e. beliefs about the major forces that determine individual health and illness. Despite the pioneering work by Saltzer (1978), it cannot be assumed that health locus of control and the behavior intentions model tap identical factors influencing a given behavior; it may well be the case there is merely some overlap. It is thus necessary to pose a question for each model.

Type and incidence of patient teaching are specified as variables for the following reasons. (1) There are multiple reasons nurses may teach in direct response to the multiple learning needs of patients. Identification of the type of teaching thus becomes important in determining relationship to health locus of control. (2) Incidence of teaching may fluctuate with the type of teaching done. It is important to separate the two components to determine accurately the relationship to health locus of control. (3) Data gathered regarding type and incidence, regardless of relationship to health locus of control will be of assistance in describing current teaching practices. There is only a relatively small amount of information available on this subject.

*Rationale for Question II: Relationship Between
Behavioral Intentions and Patient Teaching*

The reasons given above for specifying type and incidence of patient teaching also apply to Question II as do the reasons for separating the two concepts for individual consideration.

*Rationale for Question III: Relationship Between
Health Locus of Control and Behavioral Intentions*

Ideas grow and become refined through comparison and empirical testing. The two frameworks used in combination may be more powerful in describing or predicting a given behavior. Before this can take place, however, preliminary work needs to be done on the potential relationship between the two. Models combine, develop and become more complete when this type of examination is undertaken.

The three research questions may be schematically presented as illustrated in Figure 1.1.

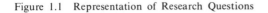
Figure 1.1 Representation of Research Questions

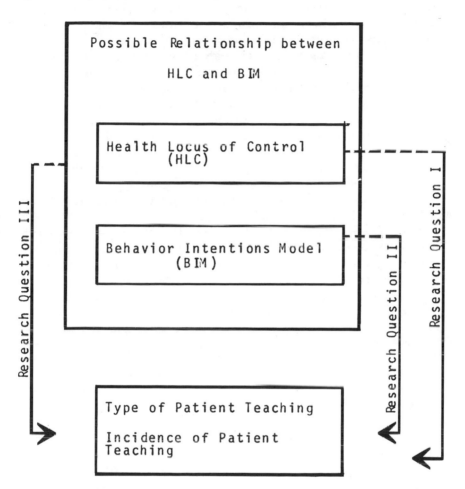

Definitions of Terms

The following definitions will be used in this study.

General hospital. General hospitals are health care agencies whose primary responsibilities are to provide acute care to any consumer. This care often requires specialized equipment or personnel in response to the onset or exacerbation of some disease.

Registered nurse-graduate nurse. A graduate nurse is defined as one who has graduated from a state approved course of nursing studies in any of the following institutions: junior college, hospital or senior college. Length of study may be as little as two years (junior college) or as many as four to five years (senior college). All nursing graduates are eligible to take the registered nurse licensure examination upon graduation.

A registered nurse is a graduate of a state approved course of nursing study who has met the licensure requirements of the state including successful completion of the state board examination.

Patient Teaching. Patient teaching is defined as a series of activites, including assessment of patients' learning needs, readiness and abilities, planning of appropriate educational strategies and programs, implementation of instructional approaches and evaluation of learning gains. The purposes of patient teaching may be to promote optimum health, prevent complications and/or encourage therapeutic processes.

Patient. Patient is defined as any person over the age of nineteen who is admitted to the hospital.

Type of Teaching. There have been many uses of the word "type" with respect to teaching. Some education authors have used the word to describe a taxonomy of teaching related to a taxonomy of learning objectives, i.e. psychomotor, cognitive or affective teaching. In the nursing literature there has been some tendency toward labeling teaching type by illness or pathology (for example, diabetic teaching) or by developmental target (for example, antenatal teaching). The word has also been used to refer to teaching methods (for example, demonstration, lecture, role playing). None of these definitions individually can cover the scope of teaching activity on a general hospital unit where there are many illnesses and developmental groups and where numerous teaching modalities may be used to meet objectives of a varied nature.

Another way to define "type" has been suggested by Redman (1976). She has described three types of teaching needs: acute, preventative and maintenance. She has suggested them as a basis for analysis of nurses' teaching patterns. These "types" are helpful in their applicability to a wide variety of patients but, at times, the categories are not mutually exclusive.

Another possible approach to "type" is via the content to be covered. Sorensen and Luckmann (1979) list twelve general areas about which patients may need to learn. These range from the cost of care to the normal anatomy and physiology of the body. If this were to be used as a typology, specificity would be gained but it would also be unwieldy to score. Statistical analysis would be limited unless a very large sample were obtained. This approach would also limit the definition of teaching to the giving of information.

Each of these approaches obviously provides information that others do not. Considering the definition of patient teaching already presented, the purpose of the study and the various possible approaches, "type" is defined on the basis of teaching activities as those activities apply to the following areas of organization of learning needs:

Type 1—Patient teaching (as defined earlier) that concerns familiarization with the hospital environment, policies and personnel.

Type 2—Patient teaching that concerns current disease state, pathology, symptoms, diagnostic tests, professionally administered therapy and prognosis.

Type 3—Patient teaching that concerns improvement/maintenance of general health including normal anatomy and physiology, sound health practices and general preventative measures.

Type 4—Patient teaching that concerns self-care, management of current illness at home (including adjustment of activities of daily living and life style) and self-administered preventative/rehabilitation measures.

These four types might be called, respectively, immediate environmental, professional management, general health and self-management teaching.

Incidence. Incidence is defined in terms of total number of patient teaching events, the number of events per patient and the amount of time spent in patient teaching.

Health locus of control. The health locus of control concept is that developed by Wallston and Wallston and is based on Rotter's social learning theory. The theory states that the potential for behavior in any specific psychological situation is a function of the expectancy of receiving a valuable reinforcement in that situation. According to the work of Wallston and Wallston, reinforcement may be seen to be under the control of the individual (internal) or under the control of outside forces such as fate or powerful others (external). This is referred to as the internal-external locus of control. When health is the focus, there is greater specificity, thus leading to the use of the term "health locus of control."

Behavior intentions model. The model is defined as that presented by Fishbein and Ajzen in 1975. According to the model, the two major factors determining behavior intentions are attitudes toward the behavior and subjective normative beliefs. The relative importance of these two components will vary depending on the individual, situation and defined behavior.

Assumptions

Assumptions for this study include:

1. The instruments will be sensitive enough to measure the specified variables.

2. Subjects will answer honestly.
3. Findings will be similar to those in other settings which use the same nursing model and serve the same patient needs.
4. Patients on medical-surgical units require teaching by registered nurses.

The first and second asumptions are presented in view of the state of the art of methodology for evaluating beliefs, attitudes and locus of control. As demonstrated in later chapters, the instruments chosen are the best currently available. None of the instruments, however, has been constructed to circumvent deliberate falsification of answers.

The third assumption is necessary because there are few existing data to suggest the applicability of variables to a wide variety of settings where the nursing role might be very different. The setting used for the study was a large suburban general hospital which has a primary care/modular approach to nursing care. The level of care and types of patient and nurse should be comparable to those in other settings with similar nursing models and geographic locations.

Finally, for the study to investigate the behavior "patient teaching," there must be some need for education on the part of the patients. A review of the research literature (Sackett, 1975) supports this as a reasonable assumption. Legal and ethical imperatives alone point to such a need.

Limitations of the Study

The study is limited to registered nurses in one hospital setting. Generalization beyond this setting may not be warranted.

The nurses were observed only during the first half of a day shift which was at least their second consecutive day on duty. The time frame was chosen because the day shift is usually the best staffed and much of the responsibility for teaching is left to the day nurse. This period is a small segment of the twenty-four hour per day care given by registered nurses. There may be large fluctuations in the type of care given and teaching done during other periods. Ascertaining that all subjects were observed on at least their second consecutive day on duty avoids the problem that nurses on medical-surgical units often encounter after time off, i.e. having to assess all new patients. Results might be different if nurses were included who were meeting all their patients initially. Findings are thus applicable only to the time frame and assignment pattern described above. The study was open only to nurses in acute care (non-intensive care) medical-surgical units who had a regular assignment to the area. Results may not be generalized beyond this parameter.

Finally, there are two other areas which must be considered when analyzing the results. First, multiple variables are examined but sample size may restrict the power of analysis in certain situations. (This will be further discussed in Chapter 4.) Second, in the strictest definition of "limitation," the findings are also limited to nurses being observed by a nurse-researcher.

The study is essentially a descriptive work which examines the relationships between teaching and specified psychological constructs. Results may be used to formulate future studies but contribute little beyond a methodological framework.

2

Conceptual Frameworks

Locus of Control

Health locus of control is a construct derived from Rotter's social learning theory. This theory proposes that "the potential for a behavior to occur in any specific psychological situation is a function of the expectancy that the behavior will lead to a particular reinforcement in that situation and the value of the reinforcement" (Rotter, 1975, p. 57). The generalized expectancy that reinforcment is under the control of the individual (internal) or outside forces such as fate, luck, chance or powerful others (external) is referred to as the internal-external locus of control (Fishbein and Ajzen, 1975). Locus of control related to health behaviors is termed health locus of control. Theoretically, knowledge of health locus of control and of values should thus help predict health behavior.

It is important to emphasize that Rotter himself does not see locus of control as the central concept of his theory. He has stated: "The nature of the reinforcement itself, whether positive or negative; the past history, sequence and patterning of such reinforcements; and the value attached to the reinforcement are obviously important and probably more crucial determinants of behavior" (Rotter, 1975, p. 56-57). Rotter proposed that social learning theory attempts to integrate reinforcement theories and cognitive-field theories.

There are four classes of variables in social learning theory: behaviors, expectancies, reinforcements and psychological situations. All four variables need to be considered, according to Rotter. He has outlined several approaches for this consideration. To predict behavior completely, expectancy, value of the reinforcement and the psychological situation would be assessed. To further complicate the problem, psychological situation may determine both expectancies and reinforcement values. For example, to predict student participation in a demonstration, it is not sufficient to determine locus of control. Available alternative activities must also be known. The psychological situation will directly affect perception of these activities.

Finally, anyone considering using locus of control must be aware of major problems often associated with its conceptualization (Rotter, 1975). The first of these is failure to treat reinforcement value as a separate variable. One should either control reinforcement value (rarely possible) or measure it (difficult but possible). For example, a health locus of control internal person may not perform regular dental hygiene simply because he does not enjoy the feel of dental floss or because he feels his best interest lies in other activities.

A second possible problem is that of specificity-generality. This has often been a problem in trying to relate locus of control to achievement behavior or performance in achievement situations, in other words, trying to predict achievement by the use of generalized expectancy of locus of control. It must be remembered that the relative importance of generalized expectancy goes up as the situation is more novel or ambiguous and goes down as the individual's experience in that situation increases. Many of the achievement situation studies using locus of control have not been novel.

Finally, there is the problem in conceptualization that the "good-bad" dichotomy might arise. It appears that internality has been equated by many people with adjustment, liberality, efficiency and social ease. This, as Rotter, Phares and others have noted, is not necessarily the case (Phares, 1976). In reality there may be situations in which "externality" is an advantage. There are often very real limits on personal control and greater trauma can result when this lack of control manifests itself via plane crashes, bankruptcies and fatal illnesses. Any study using the locus of control construct must avoid "pre-labeling" some valued behavior as internal.

Fishbein and Ajzen's Behavior Intentions Theory

In the study of health and illness, discrepancies in prediction have been noted when only the locus of control construct has been used. Often the reinforcement value has not been measured. This reinforcement value might be one of the influences on intentions to perform a given behavior. It thus appears that investigation incorporating the study of intentions would be useful. One social psychology framework is the model of behavior intentions (Fishbein and Ajzen, 1975). This model proposes that there are two factors determining behavioral intentions: (1) a personal factor which includes attitudes towards a behavior and (2) a social factor which includes subjective normative beliefs. These two factors may be given empirical weights.

Fishbein and Ajzen's views may be written as the following equation:

$$BI = (A_B) \ W_1 + (SN) \ W_2$$

BI is the intention to perform some behavior *B;* A_B is the personal attitude toward performing the behavior *B;* *SN* is the social subjective norm and W_1 and W_2 are empirically determined measures of relative importance. W_1 and W_2 will vary depending on the person, situation and behavior (Fishbein and Ajzen, 1975).

The variables that contribute to the behavioral intentions must be determined. The behavior intentions model proposes:

$$A_B = \sum_{i-1}^{n} b_i e_i$$

where *b* is the belief that performing *B* leads to consequence or outcome *i; e* is the person's evaluation of outcome *i;* and *n* is the number of beliefs the person holds about doing behavior *B*.

The second component, *SN*, might be presented as:

$$SN = \sum_{i=1}^{n} b_i m_i$$

Where b_i is the normative belief; m_i is the motivation to comply with referent *i* and *n* is the number of relevant referents (Fishbein and Ajzen, 1975).

Alternately, thoughts on the subjects may be represented schematically (Figure 2.1). Beliefs, in this system, are probability judgments, i.e. is the existence of the concept probable or improbable? Behaviors are observed acts. Behavioral intentions refer to the individual's intention to engage in various behaviors.

From this base, Fishbein and Ajzen propose that beliefs begin the chain of events which lead to behaviors. They argue that variables such as personality traits influence intentions only indirectly by influencing either the personal or social component or the relative weights of the two components. Looked at in these terms, locus of control would influence behavioral intentions by altering the importance of the personal and social factors. From the view of Rotter's social psychology, Fishbein and Ajzen's formulations are attempts to study the relationship of expectancies and certain reinforcements to behaviors. Fishbein has written:

> Fishbein's model is concerned with the relations of beliefs to attitudes, and it is of interest to note that other theorists have arrived at similar formulations in attempts to account for overt behaviors. The theories presented by Tolman, Rotter, Atkinson and others may be viewed in this light. (Fishbein and Ajzen, 1975, p. 30)

Figure 2.1   The Behavior Intentions Model*

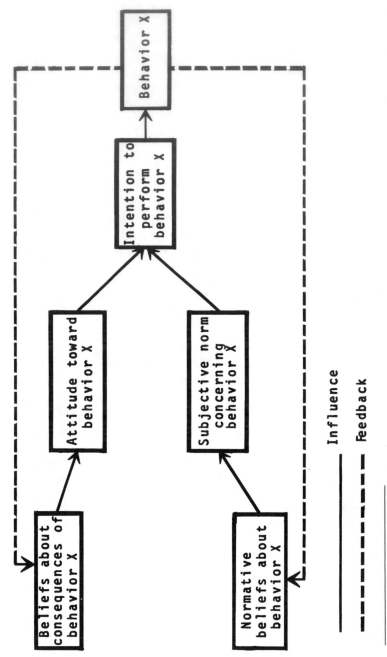

*Fishbein/Ajzen, BELIEF, ATTITUDE, INTENTION AND BEHAVIOR, © 1975, Addison-Wesley, Reading, MA. Figure 1.2. Reprinted with permission.

Frameworks and Limitations

Both theoretical frameworks described above carefully list factors which might interfere with accurate prediction or explanation of observed behavior. Some of these factors may be measured and thus included in any consideration of observed behavior. Those factors which Fishbein and Ajzen have suggested as interfering with the relationship between statement of intention and observation of behavior are the sequence of events necessary to perform the behavior, dependence on others in order to perform the behavior and lack of ability or resources. In this study, some of these factors including resources, ability and sequence will be documented.

Rotter as well as Wallston and Wallston have placed several qualifiers on the usefulness of locus of control scales (Rotter, 1975). Beyond Rotter's conceptual warnings listed earlier in this chapter, there are problems associated with the measurement of individual differences. The Rotter I-E scale has usually been used to measure locus of control. As an additive scale it has not had as high internal consistency as a power scale. As a forced choice method it does allow some control over social desirability. These measures may change, however, under different testing conditions. In other words, the scale upon which locus of control is most often tested is subject, as are all personality measures, to the conditions of testing and the conscious or unconscious purposes of the subject. Finally, there is the tendency of researchers to use a median split to obtain "internals" and "externals." Since the scale was first used, the mean score has risen from around eight ($SD = 4.0$) to ten and twelve. The distribution has always tended to be normal. Considering today's scores, early subjects once considered externals would now be labeled internals. A typology approach must definitely be avoided (Rotter, 1975).

In their consideration of this problem, Wallston and Wallston urged measuring social desirability and developing separate locus of control scales for specific dimensions of locus of control. This approach has resulted in better prediction of behavior relevant to health (Wallston et al., 1978).

A second problem has been debate over the unidimensionality versus multidimensionality of locus of control. Factor analysis by MacDonald (1973), Phares (1976), Levenson (1973, 1974, 1975) and others has fueled this argument in that early studies produced a factor analysis of a first factor of almost entirely externally worded items. Levenson argued that explanation and prediction could be improved by examining chance expectations separately from expectations influenced by powerful others. Levenson's work also supported the argument that locus of control scales worded to refer to people in general have less predictive power than personally worded items.

Other authors have rejected the multidimensionality of the construct, citing the moderate intercorrelation (r=.59) of the Levenson Powerful Other and Chance Scales. Rotter has argued that the either/or approach is contrary to a "social learning approach to the nature of stable behavior" (Rotter, 1975). The "true" structure of the construct is not revealed but the "kinds of similarities perceived by a particular group of subjects for a particular selection of items" are detailed.

Wallston and Wallston (1978), basing their work on Levenson's approach, developed a multidimensional health locus of control scale. There were very low positive correlations with appropriate internal, powerful other and chance scales. Wallston and Wallston accepted this as initial evidence of multidimensional construct validity. Definitive work on this problem is yet to be done. The present study uses the multidimensional approach because it appears reliable and logical predictions can better be made via the multidimensional approach.

A third problem has been interpreting the meaning of externality. Logically, a person who feels control is outside his own forces would be passive, unambitious, unlikely to take action. This belief has not been validated by research. Some authors (Phares et al., 1976) have attempted to identify "defensive" and "congruent" externals. The "defensive externals" are those who take action and the "congruent" are those who follow the "logical" inactive pattern. This approach has yielded very mixed results. A more productive approach might be to look at the value of the reinforcement to the person who scores as highly external.

The Study's Approach

Both frameworks have many self-admitted limitations. In Chapter 3, some other limitations will become apparent. To answer the study's central question, information (such as education, time, interruptions and reinforcers) found useful in previously cited studies of nurses and patient teaching will be gathered. This information will be correlated and analyzed with data produced via measurement of health locus of control and the behavior intentions model.

The locus of control framework as described by Wallston and Wallston emphasizes specificity. The health locus of control scale is theoretically to be related to health behavior. The behavior of teaching patients about health might then be argued to have a teaching locus of control. In other words, there may be a sound conceptual argument that despite possible strong belief in ability to control one's own health, this might not extend to taking action (teaching about health) to enable others to control their own health. Desire to control patients was one factor cited for failure to teach but no one has investigated nurses' personal health expectancies (Redman, 1976). If the nurse scores high on "chance" external orientation, will she be likely to teach? The locus of control measurement in this study thus is a contributor to what might be called the psychological situation in classic social learning theory.

The measurement of the personal and social factors of the behavior intentions model (BIM) are all related to teaching behavior. In examining the relationship of the health locus of control concept and the behavior intentions model, both the case of the differential importance of these two factors in relation to locus of control and the case of the two factors as reinforcement values will be examined.

3

Review of the Literature

In the literature concerning the behavior intentions model, health locus of control and patient teaching, there has been a variety of approaches, controversies and results. In the locus of control studies, there appears to have been some confusion about limitations of the construct and the theory from which it stems. Researchers concerned with the behavior intentions model have found problems beyond those cited by Fishbein and Ajzen. As noted earlier, patient teaching studies have also suffered from methodological and theoretical flaws.

This chapter focuses on the evolution of the health locus of control construct and the behavior intentions model. It also presents representative research approaches, methods and sources of discrepancies in findings. Where possible, emphasis is placed on studies relating the models to one another.

The Behavior Intentions Model

The behavior intentions model was proposed by Fishbein in the 1960's as an outgrowth of psychological studies of attitude. In 1968 Dulany presented an approach to behavioral prediction based on intention. In 1975 Fishbein and Ajzen presented in formal fashion the conceptual framework known as the behavior intentions model (BIM) and attempted to illustrate how the preceding diverse theoretical and empirical literature in the area could be understood within their theoretical structure. Empirical support for the model to that date is cited in that work. It is appropriate to begin the review with an examination of these studies. (A review of some of these studies also appeared in Ajzen and Fishbein, 1973.)

Research in predicting behavioral intentions has been productive when the BIM formula was used. An example of one such study was assessment of intentions of alcoholics to sign for alcoholic treatment (McArdle, 1972). The researcher obtained attitudes of subjects about signing for treatment; the subjects' normative beliefs about their spouse, doctor, parents, clergyman and significant others' views of signing for treatment as well as their motivation to comply with each of these five referents. The multiple correlation of A_B and SN (obtained by summing over the referent products) on intentions was found to be .740.

Fishbein and Ajzen (1975) cited thirteen studies as supporting their method of predicting behavioral intentions. These studies are presented in Table 3.1. Research involving determination of relative weight of attitudinal normative components concluded that, as predicted by the model, the weights vary with the behavior. There is a slight tendency for the attitude factor weight to be greater than the subjective normative factor weight. The prediction of individual differences in regression weights has also been largely supported (Fishbein and Ajzen, 1975).

Fishbein found evidence for individual differences in regression weights when undergraduate students were polled on intention to engage in premarital sexual intercourse and on the normative beliefs of families and friends. Attitudinal factors were more important than normative factors for female students. Male students were just the opposite (Fishbein and Ajzen, 1975).

Carlson (1968) reported differences in weights as a function of the kind of behavior under consideration. In a similar vein, Glassman reported that the weights of both factors varied with the target of the intention (as cited by Fishbein and Ajzen, 1975).

Buying intentions of consumers for eight different products were measured. Attitudinal considerations were the more important determinant of all eight buying intentions but subjective normative factors significantly influenced intention to buy coffee and gas.

Table 3.1.   Pertinent Studies of Intention

Study	Intention
Fishbein (1966)	Engage in premarital sexual intercourse
Carlson (1968)	Act towards African Negro
Ajzen, Fishbein (1969)	Perform leisure activities
Fishbein and others (1970)	Send communications to co-workers
Hornik (1970)	Maintain missles in game
Ajzen, Fishbein (1970)	Choose alternative in game
Ajzen (1970)	Choose alternative in game
De Vries, Ajzen (1971)	Cheat in college
Darroch (1971)	Sign photograph releases
Ajzen, Fishbein (1972)	Perform risk behavior
Jaccard, Davidson (1972)	Use birth control
McArdle (1972)	Sign for alcoholic treatment
Glassman (1971)	Buy eight products

Situational characteristics are another influence on the relative weights. One example of situational characteristics studies is the cooperative versus competitive situation. Differences due to changes in these situational characteristics were reported by Ajzen and Fishbein using gaming technique (1975).

The model's definitions for the determinants of the attitudinal and normative components have been examined extensively since the late 1960's. The attitudinal component has been examined more often than the subjective normative. Some of the studies of the attitudinal factor have included Jaccard and Davidson's (1972) investigation of family planning behaviors, McArdle's (1972) study of alcoholic behavior change. Two studies that presented empirical evidence for the formulation of subjective norms were those by King and Jaccard, and Glassman and Buckmore (as cited by Fishbein and Ajzen, 1975).

A more controversial research area for testing the model is the problem of possible effects of "external" variables. Fishbein has stated that any variable other than A_B or SN can influence behavior only indirectly (Fishbein and Ajzen, 1975). He and Ajzen have cited the studies on individual differences, type of behavior, target of intention and situational characteristics which are described above as supporting this claim (Ajzen and Fishbein, 1977).

Bentler and Speckart (1979) presented what was perhaps the first attempt to evaluate the entire model in a relatively natural context. Using three replications of a structural equation model, to represent Fishbein and Ajzen's framework, the researchers enlisted 228 college students to participate in a panel study in which attitudes, subjective norms, intentions and behaviors toward drug and alcohol use were measured. The models were rejected by goodness of fit tests but a generalized attitude-behavior model did fit data accurately. It appeared that intentions may be directly influenced by factors other than attitudes and subjective norms, i.e. previous behavior. It was also found that the effects of attitudes and previous behavior are not necessarily mediated by intentions. The authors proposed an alternate model.

Although further research may support this model, there are several flaws within the study. For example, the situation was hardly "natural." Students participated as a requirement of their introductory psychology classes and were asked to report on attitudes and behaviors such as drinking, smoking marijuana and taking cocaine, LSD and Quaaludes. The veracity of the attitude and subjective norm as well as the self-reported behaviors seems suspect. Additionally, the forces Fishbein and Ajzen cite as indirect influence (time, instability of intentions and limited degree of volitional control) may also have been at work (Fishbein and Ajzen, 1975).

In 1977 Jaccard and King proposed an alternative to Fishbein and Ajzen's formulation of the relationship between behavioral intentions and beliefs. In Jaccard and King's formulation a behavioral intention does not differ in structure from a belief but possesses the additional characteristics of linking person to action, referring person to action, and usually correlating with overt behavior. Jaccard and King analyzed behavioral intentions and proposed the following equation:

$$P_I = P_B \, P_{I\,|\,\bar{B}} + (1-P_B) \, B_{I\,|\,\bar{B}}$$

Where P_I equals intention to perform a behavior, P_B equals perceived probability that Proposition B is true, $P_{I\,|\,\bar{B}}$ equals a person's perceived probability that he would perform the behavior given that Proposition B is true, and $P_{I\,|\,\bar{B}}$ equals a person's perceived probability that he would perform the behavior given that Proposition B is not true.

This model has some obvious relations to Fishbein and Ajzen's. In several studies this model had some success (Jaccard and King, 1977; Jaccard et al., 1979). For example, in the 1979 report, there was an average correlation of .75 between predicted and obtained voting behavior. The mean correlation between predicted and obtained voting intention was .84. The computational methods available to this model (one of the conditional probabilities) would seem to circumvent many of the problems associated with the traditional regression analysis available to the behavior intentions model.

It must, however, be kept in mind that the Jaccard-King model contains many of the same elements of the behavior intentions model. Neither model appears superior in the total prediction and explanation of behavior. Both appear to achieve fairly high results but the behavior intentions model profits from repeated study. Finally, no large scale study directly comparing the two models (as in the Bentler-Speckart case) has been presented.

In 1979, Davidson and Jaccard reported a three wave, two year longitudinal study of birth control practices among 244 married women in an attempt to identify factors which moderate the attitude-behavior relation (Davidson and Jaccard, 1979). In this study Jaccard returned to the Fishbein model of behavior intentions. As is predicted by the behavior intentions model, the relations between behavior and both intention and the model's attitudinal and subjective normative factors were attenuated by (1) events in the behavioral sequence not under the volitional control of the subject, (2) an increase in the time intervals between the measurement of attitudes and behaviors and (3) changes in attitudinal and normative components during the year. Education, as is consistent with the behavior intentions model, did not affect the results.

After this study was completed, debate on the behavior intentions model centered around the definitions and operationalization of concepts. Miniard and Cohen presented results from a marketing experiment in which subjects were asked to play the role of a hypothetical female dress purchaser in responding to a questionnaire (Miniard and Cohen, 1981). Attitude toward object, referent influence potential and motivation to comply specificity were factors manipulated to allow an examination of the validity and independence of the attitudinal and normative influences on intentions. The researchers presented their findings as supporting the thesis that the model is inappropriate in distinguishing between personal and normative reasons for engagings in a specific behavior.

In a response, Fishbein and Ajzen discussed several discrepancies in Miniard and Cohen's application of the behavior intentions model which lead them to reject the study as a threat to construct validity (Fishbein and Ajzen, 1981). Although questions regarding the level at which to assess the constructs were raised, Fishbein and Ajzen noted that they believed any given manipulation could not be predefined as affecting attitudinal or normative factors. They pointed out that this is an empirical question. They also stated that the model is not truly tested if the definition of attitude is changed or if behavior intention model measures are used to measure personal and social influence instead of attitude and subjective norm.

It appears that the behavior intentions model has a great deal to offer researchers interested in the relationship of intentions, beliefs, attitudes and behaviors. There may be more models appearing in the future which allow for greater statistical freedom. There may well be models which can better position and explain what the behavior intentions model currently calls indirect influences.

This belief appears to be shared by others. As the present study was completed, a study on physician beliefs as predictors of clinical intention was reported (Cohen et al., 1980). Normative beliefs regarding vigorous diabetic management were associated with intentions to perform certain behaviors necessary in the care of the diabetic patient. The authors proposed a three year study to investigate if physicians' intentions predict clinical action and if beliefs can be used to predict or alter intentions. This long term study should contribute to an understanding of many of the issues raised by the work presented here.

For the present, the behavior intentions model appears most useful to the researcher with a cognitive-behavioral philosophy who wishes to investigate specific, well defined behaviors.

Locus of Control

There have been over 700 published articles on the concept of locus of control. There have also been many unpublished studies, master's theses and doctoral dissertations. In an area so large, there have also been several reviews and bibliographies. Among these are those by Joe (1971), Phares (1973–76) and Throop and McDonald (1971). Chapter 2 of the present study presented the chief problems researchers have had in understanding and conceptualizing the construct and the misuses and limitations associated with measurement.

It is the purpose of this section to explore in some depth the literature relating locus of control and health and illness behavior.

Health and Illness and the Locus of Control Construct

In the area of health care, the issues of control and beliefs about control become concrete. People can do a great deal to promote or disregard their health. It is obvious that the average American bombarded by the media has a relatively large body of cognitive knowledge regarding specific health practices. Smoking, drinking and the use of seat belts are just a few examples of areas in which the public has been exposed to factual health care content, yet lung cancer, alcoholism and trauma continue to be problems. Researchers have been led to ask, can health behavior be explained by individuals' beliefs about the influence their behaviors have on their health (Wallston and Wallston, 1978, p. 101)? In other words, is locus of control, as described, a predictor of health behavior?

Foremost among current researchers in this area are K. A. Wallston and B. S. Wallston. These workers have been encouraged by Strickland's 1973 report on the relationship between a belief in internal control and physical health and by research reported at the 1975 National Heart and Lung Institute Working Conference on Health Behavior. Several reports indicated a correlation between degree of internality-externality and compliance with therapeutic suggestions. Rosenstock noted that external control "is associated with higher rates of morbidity, lower rates of compliance, lower health motivation, reduced ability to control weight, smoking and use of alcohol and other drugs" (Weiss, 1975, p. 135).

Wallston and Wallston completed an extensive review of the literature in 1978 and their format will be used in this part of the review.

Preventative Behaviors

James et al. (1965) replicated Straits and Sechrest's finding that non-smokers were more likely to be internal. Steffy et al. (1970) and Lichtenstein and Kreutzer (1967), however, have failed to corroborate relationship between smoking and locus of control. Recently, Best (1975) has reported type of treatment to interact with locus of control in affecting outcome. In the area of smoking, results are thus uncertain to date.

Birth control is a second preventative behavior which has been scrutinized in relation to locus of control. MacDonald (1970) reported that "internal" single female college students were almost twice as likely to use contraceptives as their "external" classmates. Seeley (1976), Fisch (1974), and Gough (1973) in separate studies found no relationship between locus of control and contraceptive behavior.

Bauman and Udry (1972) found powerlessness to be a predictor of failure to regularly use birth control methods. Keller et al. (1970) found that feelings of efficacy were correlated with contraceptive use. Although these concepts appear similar to locus of control, there are no data relating them. Contraceptive research also appears to yield uncertain results regarding locus of control's ability to predict significantly and to explain behavior.

Weight loss studies by Manno and Marston (1972) have found internals to be more successful. O'Bryan (1972) found obese women to be consistently more external. Jeffrey and Christensen (1972) as cited by Wallston and Wallston found that internals were more likely to lose weight in a "willpower" diet program. Consistent with these reports two studies found internals more likely to complete a "self-control" weight reduction program (Balch and Ross, 1975) and both externals and internals to lose more weight in programs tailored to locus of control orientation (Wallston and Wallston, 1976). Obesity studies have thus been more consistently able to demonstrate a correlation between locus of control and a preventative health behavior.

Internality has also been linked to other preventative behaviors such as use of seat belts and preventative dental care (Williams, 1972). Dabbs and Kirscht (1971) conducted a motivational locus of control study on college students' inoculation against influenza. Both factors appeared predictive under different methods of analysis. As Kirscht (1972) has since pointed out, it is difficult but necessary to distinguish carefully between the two concepts in a research design.

Sick Role Behavior

Research on sick role behavior has centered around three areas: physical response to illness, information seeking behavior and compliance with selected therapeutic regimens. Johnson et al. (1970) found female internal patients who had undergone surgery received more analgesics. First born internals also had longer hospital stays.

Cromwell et al. (1977) reported that myocardial infarction patients in a "congruent" condition (internals with high participation in nursing care and externals with low participation) returned to the hospital or died within twelve weeks of discharge. During hospitalization, externals spent a larger percentage of their days in the coronary care unit and had higher temperatures and lactate dehydrogenase levels.

Internals, after initial diagnosis, appear to seek information more actively about their condition and to possess more information. This finding has been replicated despite differences in conditions (Seeman and Evans, 1962; Lowery, 1974; Lowery and DuCette, 1976). These findings have been replicated even in college student role playing situations (Wallston et al., 1976).

In illnesses short in duration with proper care, internals are more likely to return for treatments (Darrow, 1973). In illnesses of a long term nature, such as hypertension and diabetes, there appears to be no relationship between compliance and locus of control. Internals begin more compliant but under long term care become less compliant. DuCette, in the case of diabetes, has hypothesized that the unpredictable aspects and sequelae of the disease discourage internals, i.e. even perfect compliance with suggested regimens does not always lead to control. The internal patient thus shifts away from personal efforts aimed at control. Wallston and Wallston (1975) suggest such findings might also be related to failure to include measures of perceived value of health in the research design.

There is some evidence that the locus of control construct is relevant to the study of health and sick-role behaviors. There is also a disquieting lack of consistent findings. What have been some of the problems which might explain these findings?

First, many of the studies used Rotter's I-E scale instead of a more specific area locus of control scale. Potter (1975) himself has recommended that specific measures of locus of control may be valuable in predicting a specific locus of control orientation in practical situations. In the health–sick role behavior area, Wallston, et al. (1978) have developed the Health Locus of Control (HLC) and the Multidimensional Health Locus of Control (MHLC) scales. These have been found to be more accurate than the generalized I-E scale in health research. Researchers have constructed even more specific scales geared to behavior or development level. One example is Saltzer's (1978) Weight Locus of Control (WLOC) scale and another is Parcel and Mayer's Children's Health Locus of Control (CHLOC) scale. The ideal level of scale specificity has yet to be ascertained.

Second, both Rotter (1975) and Wallston et al. (1978) have emphasized that, in studies on locus of control, there must be some consideration of the value of the reinforcement which is achieved by performing a given behavior. Many of the early studies of locus of control and health behavior failed to do this.

Third, it is possible that differences in intentions to perform a given behavior may be influenced. Using the behavior intentions model, Saltzer found greater importance of social norms for externals and greater importance of personal attitudes for internals.

Fourth, many studies used the median split method of determining internality-externality, creating possibly false dichotomies.

Health Professionals' Behaviors

At the time of this study, there were no reported studies of the influence of health locus of control on the behavior of health professionals either toward their own health or toward their clients.

Patient Teaching

This section will consider some of the studies of registered nurse involvement in patient teaching as well as the implications of the reviews of health locus of control and the behavior intentions model literature.

Many of the classic reasons for a lack of patient teaching by nurses were cited in Chapter 1. As noted in that review, many of the studies which supported these reasons must now be looked at in the light of a rapidly changing professional atmosphere.

One reason for not teaching is confusion over the nurse's role. Streeter (1953) found metropolitan nurses attributed teaching about rehabilitation to the physician's or social worker's role. Malone et al. (1962) reported that only two out of ninety nurses in an outpatient setting thought the physician would ask them to teach the patients. Von Schilling (1968) reported such role uncertainty might lead to failure to teach mothers of children with defects. If the physician does not tell a mother about a defect, the nurse cannot usurp what is often the doctor's legal prerogative.

It must be noted that these studies are all very old by the profession's development clock. In 1980, however, nurses were still encountering problems with physician antagonism (McCulloch, Boggs, Varner, 1980). Despite occasional role conflicts, research has shown nurses expect to teach and often assign it a high priority (Palm, 1971).

Pohl reported that the modal nurse in her study of patient teaching had taken no courses in teaching (Pohl, 1965). One-third of the subjects reported they had no training for the teaching they were doing. Since that time, all nursing programs have included content on principles and methods of teaching and learning. Lack of teaching skill was still, however, an obstacle according to a study done in 1980 (McCulloch, Boggs, Varner, 1980). Murdaugh has presented one study of coronary care nurses in which subjects were given a course in teaching learning principles (Murdaugh, 1980). The average score on the pretest was 56%. After exposure to this course in teaching, knowledge of patients regarding their condition and care increased. It is also interesting to note that before the course, the most frequently given reasons for not teaching were lack of time, lack of patient emotional readiness, physician interference and lack of teaching skill. After the course, lack of continuity and physician interference were most often cited. Lack of ability to teach was no longer an important factor.

In a related vein, other authors have cited lack of knowledge about content as a reason for failure to teach (Redman, 1976). This was one of the top four reasons given by subjects in Streeter's study. Twenty-five years later, this possibility is still being raised by nurses investigating patient education in subject areas such as diabetes, chronic lung disease and arthritis. Scheiderich (1980) reported that only 15.9% of eighty-two medical and surgical staff nurses were able to score at or above the level necessary to teach diabetics. Although there are some questions about what knowledge is necessary to teach diabetics, this study raises disturbing questions when one considers how many different areas a registered nurse may be expected to be competent to teach.

Another reason for not teaching is lack of expectations by employers and/or a lack of staff, time or resources. In a report on implementation of an educational program, all of these problems were reported (McCulloch, Boggs and Varner, 1980). Physicians saw education programs as a threat, materials were inefficiently organized and there was a reticence to teach due to a lack of familiarity with teaching tools and methods. It was found that during periods of high census completed patient teaching dropped as low as 14%. During the lowest census month, 80% of teaching was completed. With a change in organization of teaching, completed teaching stayed around 80% even in periods of high census.

Some of the processes and solutions described in the McCulloch report mirror the developmental issues that hospitals face in providing patient education. Redman has described developmental phases and issues which influence the teaching actually done (Redman, 1981). The major issues reported include the topics of decision making, the degree of coordination and management and the requirements for demonstrating outcome and quality. It was found that five to seven years was the length of time needed for maturation in the institutions that took part in the study. Redman speculated that this period of time might be lengthy due to the structure of the health care delivery system. The non-research literature tends to support this idea. It appears that employers do expect patient teaching but that there are an even greater number of other expectations with at least equally high priority.

Finally, there have been numerous sociological articles on the use of knowledge as a commodity to be used in controlling the health practitioner–client relationship (Freidson, 1970). These ideas have not been recently tested. It appears more efforts are needed in this area to be able to comment on this idea within today's health care milieu.

In summary, many reasons for not teaching can be found within the nursing literature. For some of these reasons there has been some research support but for others there has been either mere speculation or reliance on very old data. Beyond the need for exploring some of these ideas there is also the need to investigate other possibilities.

There may be other factors influencing the occurrence of patient teaching which are yet to be explored. One of these is nurses' beliefs regarding their ability to influence health. The nurse who has a high "chance" health locus of control might be less inclined to teach. Such a finding would also open many questions regarding certain postulates of the social learning theory. Beyond this possible application of the health locus of control, there appear to be other useful avenues for investigation. In a study of patient teaching, the behavior intentions model would suggest a way not only to study the postulated relationship of employers' expectations of nurses but also to examine the influence of other personnel. Using the behavior intentions model would also enable the researcher to examine the relationship of attitudes toward patient teaching and actual teaching behavior.

4

Methodology and Procedure

Registered or graduate nurses acting as module leaders on eight medical-surgical units in a general hospital were selected as described below. Subjects were observed by the investigator on the second consecutive tour on a week day, day shift from 0700 to 1100. This observation included timing and listing each activity and message as well as the initiator and participants in each activity. The subjects were also asked to complete a questionnaire which included the health locus of control scale, items related to the behavior intentions model and demographic items. Data collection took place during the summer of 1979.

The hospital studied is a five hundred bed, voluntary teaching institution located in a large suburb of a major midwestern city. The hospital sponsors a diploma school of nursing and a medical residency program. The town in which it is located is moderately affluent. The hospital draws most of its patients from this town and surrounding suburbs.

This institution was chosen because of several advantages. The department of nursing has long been committed to patient teaching. This commitment has resulted in the nursing staff's development of specific standards for patient teaching. Although the standards are individualized for each case, there is thus some way to measure the teaching done. The department of nursing has also shown its commitment to patient teaching through the provision of multiple resources (such as audiovisuals) which are available to each unit. Each nurse is responsible for patient teaching but may call on subject specialists when necessary. In this way, the department has avoided problems that arise when only (diabetic or hypertension or other) specialists teach on their narrow subject.

The department further allows for accountability in patient care by using the modular-primary nurisng system. Registered nurses are module leaders. These modules may be as small as two or three patients or as large as eight or nine. The nurse is responsible for all nursing care. In the case of a larger module i.e. eight or nine patients, an assistant is provided. This assistant may be another registered nurse (rarely) or a practical nurse or an aide. On the day shift, there are few aides compared to most hospitals. The hospital does not have an aide training program and is attempting to implement a direct care by nurses only policy. The aides who are employed are either long time employees or nursing students on vacation.

The module is composed of all the nurse's primary patients plus some of the primary patients of nurses who are off duty. The nurse is directly responsible for developing a plan of care and providing it.

The nurses employed at this institution are most often diploma graduates. Baccalaureate graduates are the next largest group and associate degree graduates a small minority. The hospital does, however, employ a larger percentage of baccalaureate graduates than the average for the area. The presence of a diploma school on the premises and the generally higher proportion of diploma graduates in this area no doubt accounts for the preparation mix.

Only hospital approved medical-surgical units were used in the study. This resulted in a pool of eight units. Two other medical-surgical units were not used. One was not used due to administrative changes and staffing difficulties; the other was not used due to staffing problems and the general nature of patient census at the time of the study (the majority of patients were either comatose or disoriented). No acute specialty units (intensive care, burns, coronary care) or rehabilitation, isolation, pediatric, psychiatric or obstetric units were used due to anticipated wide variance between nursing activities on these units. The hospital does differentiate between medical and surgical units although surgical patients may be sent to medical units and medical patients to surgical units when bed space is limited.

One of the eight units used in the study identified itself as chiefly orthopedic. For the purpose of the study, this was considered a surgical floor. Three other units were identified as surgical units. Four units were considered medical units.

The hospital's staffing policy is that a nurse may request permanent night or afternoon duty. There is no permanent day duty available for the staff nurses on the medical-surgical units. Nurses who wish to work day shift must agree to work one other shift as needed. In practice, this means rotation to another shift at least once per month. The nurses must agree to work weekends. At the time of this study, this meant each nurse worked two out of three weekends.

Procedures and Techniques

Subject Selection and Contact

The study was limited to registered or graduate nurses eligible for licensure as registered nurses. The procedure for subject selection was to list all registered nurses on the involved medical-surgical units who would work as module leaders at least two consecutive day shifts, the second of which would be on a week day. The names were then randomly selected with replacement. Using this method, thirty-two subjects were selected. This is almost half of the eligible group.

The nurses' schedules were then checked and a list drawn up by unit as to when the randomly selected nurses would be on at least a second tour of day shift, week day duty. Prior to contacting the nurses, the permissions of both the area coordinator (supervisor) and the unit coordinator (head nurse) were obtained.

The nurse was then approached by the researcher who explained the purpose of the study as an investigation of factors influencing patient teaching. The procedure to be followed was outlined and the confidentiality of any information provided was assured. After once again reminding the nurse that participation was voluntary, the researcher asked the nurse to sign a witnessed consent form. This was in keeping with requirements for the protection of rights of human subjects.

Observation Periods

The observation periods began at 0700 and ended at 1130. Due to differences in scheduled lunch periods for nurses, usable data were gathered by observation from 0700 to 1100. The investigator accompanied the nurse during this period and on data flow sheets noted the time an activity began and ended, the activity itself, the initiator, participants and any interruptions. When the nurse interacted with a patient, the nurse's responses were noted. No inferences were made; no coding was done.

The nurse introduced the investigator to each patient as a nurse-researcher and explained the general purpose of the study as a "study of the nurses' activities during the day." The patient was then asked if the nurse-researcher might stay. No patient refused. There were, however, several times when it was deemed inappropriate by either the nurse or researcher for the investigator to accompany the nurse. These were recorded under activity as "a patient interaction."

The definition of an activity was any specific pursuit. Activities were merely recorded on the flow sheet. No attempt was made during the observation period to qualify them. The initiator was defined as the person who began an activity without the request of another. Participants were defined as anyone who took part in the activity other than the initiator. Interruption was defined as anything or anyone other than the nurse herself who broke into the continuity of an activity.

Observer Training

The use of a nonparticipant nurse observer as a data collection instrument was dictated by a desire to avoid the mere estimation by subjects of the amount of teaching done. This desire was heightened by the results of the pilot study in which potential subjects often stated they were not doing any teaching and so could not be subjects. An additional incentive to use this technique was the apparent hesitancy of potential subjects in the pilot study when informed that a tape recording would be necessary. As the study was designed, it would also have been almost impossible to preserve spontaneity if tape recording techniques were used as each person who was recorded would have had to sign a consent prior to the interaction.

Observer training took place over a week long period during which there was, at first, constant, then, random validation of the recording of activities until there were no discrepancies noted in two consecutive four hour periods.

Use of a nurse-observer offered several advantages in terms of acceptance by patients and staff. The nurses were able to proceed with their daily activities without giving continuous explanations. The nurse-observer may also have been able to tolerate some situations which would have been distracting to a non-nurse (cardiac emergencies, dressing changes). It is believed there is greater reliability in the recording of familiar events. Although these advantages have been verified by other researchers, there are also some disadvantages, chiefly decreased reliability despite reliability testing. Use of a second observer to overcome this problem was not considered worthwhile due to the increased physical and psychological crowding yet another observer would add to the situation.

Questionnaire Administration

The questionnaire was pretested as taking approximately fifteen minutes to complete. Subjects were asked to answer the questionnaire immediately after observation. In three cases, questionnaires could not be completed due to patient care responsibilities. These questionnaires were returned to the researcher the following day. No names were placed on the questionnaire.

A number was assigned to the questionnaire which matched the number assigned to the observation flow sheet. This was done to insure the possibility of correct correlation between observed behavior and questionnaire answers.

Instruments

Health Locus of Control

Each subject completed Form A of the Multidimensional Health Locus of Control (MHLC) scale as developed by Wallston and Wallston in 1978. This is an eighteen item, personally worded instrument designed to reflect three dimensions of health locus of control beliefs: internality (IHLC); powerful other (PHLC); and chance (CHLC) externality. The reading level required, calculated using the Dale-Chall formula, is between fifth and sixth grade.

The alpha reliabilities for the MHLC scale have been reported as between .673 and .767. The IHLC, PHLC and CHLC scales have been found to be statistically independent. Form A of the PHLC and CHLC scales have been reported to be slightly but not significantly correlated.

Although the scales are relatively new, they have been tested and used beyond their initial development. Wallston and Wallston (1978) reported studies in progress to attempt to meet the multitrait-multimethod approach to validation. Two alternatives reported under investigation were the self-rating task approach and the behavior simulation approach.

To put the scales in perspective, Wallston and Wallston (1978) reported exploring the possibility that yet another conceptually independent dimension may exist. This dimension revolves around environmental causes of health and illness. These causes include such factors as weather, pollution and germs. Another area that is currently being studied is the possible overlap of another orthogonal dimension (such as expectations of success-failure). Despite these areas of uncertainty it appears that the MHLC scales provide an instrument on which some estimates of validity and reliability have been established.

Behavior Intentions Model

Many researchers have used different methods to operationalize the BIM components. In general, the usual method for ascertaining the dependent variable (intention) has been to ask the subject to respond to a question regarding intent to perform a specific behavior. Measurement of the personal attitude and subjective norm, however, have not met with such universal treatment.

In some studies, including many of the earlier BIM studies, personal attitude was measured using a semantic differential tool. The use of the semantic differential appears to have several advantages in that the general personal feeling of favorableness or unfavorableness toward some stimulus may be measured for different individuals without fear that the wording of the consequences of the attitude will be so concrete as to be limiting to individual cases. Fishbein and Ajzen (1975, p. 78) note that the items with a high loading on the evaluative factor constitute a semantic differential scale for the measurement of attitude toward a concept.

Jaccard and Davidson (1972) found that the evaluative semantic differential scales were highly related to beliefs about consequences of an act and evaluation of those consequences. This later approach has since been used by many researchers. It has the advantage of specifically applying the BIM formulation that attitude is the sum of the products of the belief about consequences by evaluation of that consequence. It has the disadvantage that beliefs about consequences may be too numerous and highly subject specific if the project wishes to study any other variables. For example, Saltzer (1978) reported using twenty-four possible consequences of losing weight. Adding to this dilemma, Grotelueschen and Caulley (1977) have argued that respondents should not answer those items in which the consequence is not relevant. This practice would result in data useful only on an individual basis. For the purpose of this investigation, a four item semantic differential was used.

The normative component (SN) has typically been ascertained by summing the products of the subject's estimation of the opinion of favorability of a referent person or group times the motivation to comply with the referent. This (SN) calculation is often easier for the researcher to do if the referents are usually fewer in number and more universal in type than the consequences needed to calculate the attitude component. In pretesting it was noted that five referent groups were consistently discussed by nurses; the head nurse, fellow nurses on the unit, patients, other nurses and physicians. These five groups were thus used as referents in the construction of the subjective norm component. Following Grotelueschen and Caulley's suggestion that all groups be referents or be omitted by the respondent, it was previously ascertained that the five groups were referents to all subjects. There may, however, have been other, unmeasured, referents in individual cases.

Other Information

Subjects were asked to complete a role scale to be used in future examination of role perception's effect on teaching. Subjects were also asked to complete demographic questions including degrees held, number of years since graduation, number of years of clinical practice, the number of years in positions where patient teaching is expected, position title, unit type, years in current position, employment status, and number of years employed at hospital.

Other information collected included the ranking of facets of nursing activities in terms of importance and personal interest. Information about educational preparation for specific aspects of patient teaching was also requested in the questionnaire.

Methods of Analysis

All calculations were made using the Statistical Package for the Social Sciences (Version 8) computer program. The alpha level for significance testing was set at .05.

Observations

After all data were collected, an independent rater assessed all activity/interactions according to whether teaching, as previously defined, occurred during the interaction. The type of teaching done was also rated. The rater was a registered nurse oriented to the operational definition of teaching and the four teaching descriptions. Practice in rating activity/interactions was provided. Reliability with another rater was .98 after the training period.

An activity/interaction was rated as teaching if there was an assessment of learning needs, readiness or abilities, and/or planning of educational strategies and programs, and/or implementation of instructional approach and/or evaluation of learning progress. The activity/interaction was rated Type 1 if it aimed at teaching the patient about the hospital policies, environment or personnel. It was rated as Type 2 if it concerned the current disease, pathology, diagnostic tests, therapy or prognosis. It was rated Type 3 if it concerned improvement/maintenance of general health including sound health practices or preventative measures. It was rated Type 4 if it concerned self-care of a health problem including adjustment of activities of daily life, self-administered treatments, rehabilitative procedures or measures designed to prevent further complications. Table 4.1 lists some example activity/interactions for each type.

Health Locus of Control Scales

The health locus of control scales were analyzed following the procedure suggested by Wallston and Wallston (1978). Scores for the items applicable to each of the three scales were summed. This yielded the requisite three scores per subject: powerful other health locus of control (PHLC), chance health locus of control (CHLC) and internal health locus of control (IHLC).

Table 4.1. Example of Teaching Activity/Interactions by Type

Type 1: Teaching About Hospital and Hospital Policies

1. Tells patient about differences in duties of personnel providing care.
2. Orients patient to use of various call bells in room.

Type 2: Teaching About Disease Process and/or Therapy Administered by Health Care Personnel

1. Secures diagrams of atherosclerotic vessels to use in teaching patient about hypertension.
2. Explains chemotherapy's action on cells to cancer patient.

Type 3: Teaching Positive Health Practices

1. Discusses measures to prevent bladder infection with young woman.
2. Demonstrates proper use of tooth brush.

Type 4: Teaching Self-management at Home

1. Discusses high calorie recipes and food preparation techniques with emaciated cancer patient who is about to be discharged.
2. Has patient return demonstrate the proper application of nitro paste.

Behavior Intention Items

The attitude component of the BIM was calculated by summing the scores on the attitude semantic differential items after appropriately reversing the alternating favorableness adjectives to provide comparable scoring.

The normative component was calculated by summing the products of the estimation of the opinion of a referent towards the subject performing times the motivation to comply with the referent. This follows the standard technique specified by Fishbein and Ajzen (1975).

Demographic and Other Information

These data were coded, transferred to coding sheets for keypunching and then punched on computer cards for use in data analysis.

Appendix A includes the role scale as well as all other scales and demographic information as it was obtained from the subjects. Appendix B presents the form used in making and recording observations.

5

Results

Sample Description

Thirty-two subjects were randomly selected as described in Chapter 4. Two persons from this random selection did not take part in the study. One of these potential subjects gave no reason at the time of the refusal but changed jobs the next week. The other potential subject was not approached at the request of the head nurse. Both subjects were replaced by random drawing from the original pool.

All subjects were female. The educational characteristics of the nurses are presented in Table 5.1. The majority, nineteen (59%), were graduated from a diploma program. One-third, ten, began their careers with a baccalaureate degree; only two (7%) held the associate degree. No subject held any degree in nursing other than her original educational qualification. Seven subjects, however, held degrees in non-nursing fields. Three held the associate of arts degree, three held the bachelor of arts degree and one held a master of arts degree.

The majority of nurses reported undergraduate course content in the following areas: assessment of patient learning needs (90.9%), use and selection of audiovisual materials (75.1%), methods of classroom and group instruction (65.7%) and strategies to increase compliance with therapeutic regimens (65.6%). All nurses reported having received some type of education (undergraduate courses, postgraduate courses or continuing education programs) on assessment of patient learning needs. Two nurses indicated no education in the use and selection of audiovisual materials. Four nurses indicated no training in classroom or group instruction. Three nurses reported never having been exposed to content regarding strategies to increase patient compliance.

The employment characteristics of the sample can be seen in Table 5.2. Eighteen of the nurses were from essentially medical units and fourteen from surgical units (including orthopedics). Twenty-eight subjects held the title "staff nurse" and four held the title "nurse clinician." The title "nurse clinician" is granted at the institution to recognize clinical expertise in

Table 5.1. Education Characteristics: Frequencies and Percentages of 32 Nurses

Characteristics	F	%
Basic Nursing Education		
Diploma	19	59.4
Associate Degree	2	6.3
Baccalaureate	10	31.3
Omitted	1	3.1
Highest Nursing Education		
Original degree only	32	100
Other Education		
Associate of Arts	3	9.3
Bachelor of Arts	3	9.3
Master of Arts	1	3.1
Education for Patient Teaching		
Assessment of patient learning needs		
Undergraduate only	20	62.5
Graduate course only	1	3.1
Continuing education only	5	15.6
Undergraduate & graduate course	5	15.6
Undergraduate & continuing education	1	3.1
Undergraduate, continuing education & graduate course	2	6.3
Not at all	2	6.3
Classroom and group teaching methods		
Undergraduate only	16	50.0
Graduate course only	1	3.1
Continuing education only	2	6.3
Undergraduate & graduate course	3	9.4
Undergraduate & continuing education	6	18.8
Not at all	4	12.5
Strategies for increasing patient compliance		
Undergraduate only	17	53.1
Graduate course only	4	12.5
Continuing education only	3	9.4
Undergraduate & graduate course	3	9.4
Graduate & continuing education	1	3.1
Undergraduate, graduate and continuing education	1	3.1
Not at all	3	9.4

Table 5.2. Employment Characteristics: Frequencies and Percentages of 32 Nurses

Characteristics	F	%
Type of Unit		
Medical	18	56.3
Surgical	14	43.7
Title		
Staff nurse	28	87.5
Nurse clinician	4	12.5
Number of years at this institution		
Less than 1	12	37.5
1	13	40.6
2	3	9.4
Over 5	4	12.5
Number of years of practice		
Less than 1	7	21.9
1	9	28.1
2	8	25.0
3–5	2	6.3
Over 5	6	18.3
Hours of work		
Full time	29	90.6
Part time	3	9.4
Number of years of patient teaching		
1 or less	24	75.0
2	1	3.1
3–5	2	6.3
Over 5	4	12.5
No response	1	3.1
Number of assigned patients		
4	2	6.3
5	6	18.8
6	4	12.5
7	11	34.3
8	8	25.0
9	1	3.1
Assistants		
None	10	31.3
1	22	68.8

nursing. It is not an administrative title nor does it require formal advanced nursing education. Twenty-nine nurses were employed full time and three were employed part time. The part time subjects worked at least six out of every fourteen calendar days.

Only four nurses had been employed at the hospital for more than five years. Over three-quarters of the nurses had worked at the hospital for one year or less. Half of the nurses reported working one year or less. This is not surprising considering the typical turnover in nursing employment and the low rate at which experienced nurses desire or stay in staff positions. There is some difference between years of reported nursing practice and years in positions in which patient teaching was expected. This may be due to assignment to such areas as the operating room or recovery room. It may also be that patient teaching was not expected despite patient contact. This was more common twenty years ago and indeed the discrepancies were reported by three of the nurses having the longest professional experience.

On the day observed, ten of the subjects (31.3%) functioned alone. The majority (twenty-two or 68.8%) had an aide or licensed practical nurse for assistance. Over half of the subjects (eighteen or 56.3%) had no other duties but to care for assigned patients on the day observed. Fourteen nurses (43.8%), however, had not only to care for patients but also to act as "resource person." "Resource person" is analogous to acting as charge nurse. Responsibilities include (but are not limited to) giving report to the unit secretary, answering the questions of other personnel and reassigning personnel as needed. One subject's responsibility as resource person included orienting new nurses. The number of patients assigned varied from four to nine with seven being the mode. The mean number assigned ($\bar{X}$) was 6.6.

Rankings of the most personally enjoyable nursing activities are presented in Table 5.3. Eleven subjects rated patient observation and recording as their favored activity. Seven nurses ranked patient advocacy as their first choice. Patient teaching was ranked first by five nurses as was performing skilled procedures. Three nurses indicated coordinating and teaching other health care team members as their favorite activity. One nurse used the fill-in option to indicate helping patients adjust to illness and death and dying as the most rewarding activity.

Research Question I: What Is the Relationship Between Health Locus of Control and Type and Incidence of Patient Teaching by Registered or Graduate Nurses in a General Hospital?

Health Locus of Control

Reliability. The alpha reliabilities of the Multidimensional Health Locus of Control (MHLC) scales are: .74 Powerful Others Health Locus of Control

Table 5.3. Ranking of Nursing Activities as Personally Enjoyable: Frequencies and Percentages of 32 Nurses

Activities	F	%
Performing skilled procedures		
1	5	15.6
2	9	28.1
Coordinating and teaching other health team members		
1	3	9.4
2	1	3.1
Patient advocacy		
1	7	21.9
2	7	21.9
Patient teaching		
1	5	15.6
2	9	28.1
Patient observation and recording		
1	11	34.4
2	6	18.8
Other		
1	1	3.1
2	0	—

(PHLC), .73 Internal Health Locus of Control (IHLC) and .618 Chance Health Locus of Control (CHLC). No MHLC scale is significantly correlated with any other MHLC scale. Correlations between scales range from .2 (IHLC and CHLC) to +.2 (PHLC and CHLC).

MHLC scores. The PHLC mean is 16.06 and the standard deviation 5.43. The range is 6 to 28. The IHLC mean is 25.46 and the standard deviation is 4.07. The range is 14 to 34. The CHLC mean is 16.25 and the standard deviation 4.072. The range is 6 to 28. (The minimum score attainable on any of these scales is 6 and the maximum is 36.) Analysis of variance was done to determine the effect of level of education and years of nursing practice on the health locus of control. Neither of these variables resulted in significant differences on any of the scales.

Teaching Incidence and Type

Incidence. The different measures of teaching incidence with appropriate descriptive statistics are presented in Table 5.4. The average number of

Table 5.4.   Incidence of Patient Teaching:
Means, Standard Deviations, Ranges

Operationalization of Incidence	$\bar{X}$	S.D.	Range
Total number of teaching events	4.96	4.13	0–19
Total number minutes spent teaching	17.68	14.13	0–55
Average number of minutes per teaching event	3.78	2.04	0–9
Number of teaching events per patient	.45	.59	0–4

teaching events is 4.96 per nurse with a very wide range of 0 to 19. In only one case did no teaching occur. The average amount of time spent teaching was 17.7 minutes. This is approximately 7% of the 240 minutes of observed nursing time per subject. The average time nurses spent in morning report was 28 minutes. If this is omitted on the grounds it is nondiscretionary time, the average percentage of time spent teaching rises to 8%. Total teaching time was correlated with number of teaching events (.766, $p < .01$).

Figures 5.1 and 5.2 present the distribution of teaching incidence as measured in total number of minutes and total events. Six to eight minutes is the most frequently occurring total number of minutes taught with seven nurses in this category. Three nurses taught from zero to two minutes total. Six nurses, however, taught for over a half-hour. The total number of teaching events is bimodal at two and three events. Fourteen of the subjects are accounted for in these categories. One nurse had nineteen teaching events recorded.

Type. Table 5.5 presents the incidence of types of teaching events with appropriate descriptive statistics. Type 2 was most frequent with an average incidence per nurse of 2.72. Types 1, 3 and 4 occurred on the average less than one time per observation period. The means for these types were, respectively, .63, .82 and .94. In the case of Type 1 teaching the standard deviation is small (.71). Types 2, 3 and 4 have larger standard deviations (2.88, 1.91 and 1.11, respectively). The greatest range of incidence is seen with Type 2. One nurse was observed in fourteen separate Type 2 teaching incidents. In considering length of time for each type incident, Type 4 teaching produced the longest average incident ($\bar{X}$ = 4 minutes) while Type 1 produced the shortest ($\bar{X}$ = less than 1 minute).

Some of the teaching types showed almost no variation. Incidence of teaching types is over 75% accounted for by a range of 0 (zero) to 2. This lack of variability, especially in Type 1 teaching, requires careful consideration when interpreting correlational analysis (Table 5.6).

No teaching type was significantly correlated with any other teaching

Figure 5.1. Minutes Spent Teaching for 32 Nurses

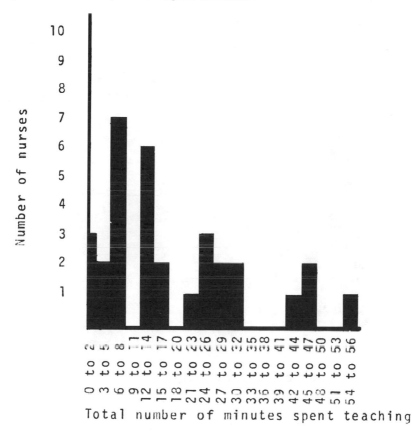

type with the exception of the correlation between Type 1 and 3 which was .42 ($p < .01$).

Relationship between health locus of control and incidence and type of teaching. The nature and size of the relationship between two variables may be measured by a correlation coefficient. Considering the nature of the data and the lack of an explicit hypothesis concerning the direction of the coefficient, the Pearson product moment correlation coefficient with a two-tailed test of significance was applied. Table 5.7 presents the coefficients. All correlations are low and nonsignificant with the exception of the correlations between Type 4 teaching and the IHLC and CHLC scales. In the former case there appears to be a moderately positive correlation (.38) and in the latter case there appears to be a moderately negative correlation (-.40).

The product moment correlation coefficient is a measure of goodness of

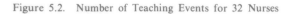

Figure 5.2. Number of Teaching Events for 32 Nurses

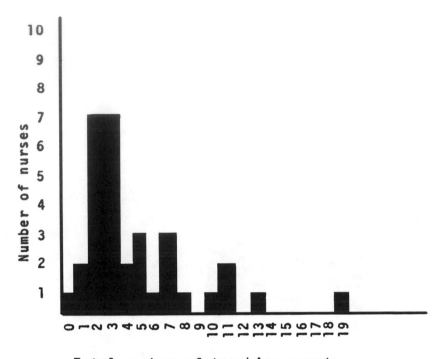

Table 5.5. Incidence of Teaching Types:
Means, Standard Deviations, Ranges

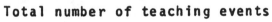

Teaching Types	$\overline{X}$	S.D.	Range
Teaching about hospital policy, etc.	.625	.707	0–2
Teaching about current disease pathology, diagnostic tests, professionally administered treatment	2.719	2.876	0–14
Teaching about positive health practices, prevention measures	.813	1.908	0–10
Teaching about self-care & management of disease at home	.938	1.105	0–4

Table 5.6. Frequency of Teaching Type for 32 Nurses

Teaching Type	Frequency
Type 1. Teaching about Hospital Policy, etc.	
None	15
1 or 2 Events	17
Type 2. Teaching about Current Disease, Professionally Administered Treatments	
None	2
1 or 3 Events	23
3 or More	7
Type 3. Teaching about Positive Health Practices	
None	23
1 or 2 Events	8
3 or More	3
Type 4. Teaching about Self-Care at Home	
None	14
1 or 2 Events	13
3 or More	4

Table 5.7. Product Moment Correlations Between Multidimensional Health Locus of Control Scales and Incidence and Type of Patient Teaching

Patient Teaching Incidence & Type of Patient Teaching	Multidimensional Health Locus of Control Scales		
	PHLC	IHLC	CHLC
Total number of teaching events	.20	.09	.02
Total minutes spent teaching	.20	.13	−.06
Type 1	.09	.02	−.10
Type 2	.13	.07	.12
Type 3	.28	−.12	.11
Type 4	.08	.38*	−.40*

Note: A two-tailed test of significance was used.
*$p < .05$

fit for a linear regression line. Relationships may also be curvilinear. Scattergrams constructed for each of the possible relationships failed to indicate such a property. Polynomial regression was thus considered unwarranted.

Summary. The Multidimensional Health Locus of Control scales and incidence and type of teaching behaviors appear to be statistically unrelated with the exception of a correlation between Type 4 teaching and IHLC (.38) and a negative correlation between Type 4 and CHLC (–.40).

Research Question II: What is the Relationship Between the Variables of the Behavior Intentions Model and the Type and Incidence of Teaching Done by Registered or Graduate Nurses in a General Hospital?

Attitudes

The alpha reliability of the attitude scale is .786. Attitude scores (A) for the behavior of patient teaching were computed as described in Chapter 4. The maximum achievable score would thus be 12 (positive attitude) and the minimum –12 (negative attitude). A neutral score would be zero and indicate a neutral attitude. The mean A score is 10.8 with a standard deviation of 2.29. The range is –1 to +12. Analysis of variance was performed. There is no significant difference in attitude based on education or years of nursing practice.

Subjective Norm

The alpha reliability of the subjective norm is .735. Subjective norm (SN) scores for the behavior of patient teaching were computed as described in Chapter 4. The maximum achievable score would thus be 245 and the minimum score would be 5. The mean SN score is 164.84 with a standard deviation of 51.59. The range is 82 to 238.

Analysis of variance was performed. There is no significant difference in SN scores based on education or years of nursing practice.

Behavioral Intentions

The mean behavioral intention (BI) is 5.62 with a standard deviation of 1.28. The range is 3 to 7. Overall mean rating of behavioral intention to teach is lower than the mean rating of the importance of teaching (6.53 and .717). Rating of the importance of teaching and BI are significantly correlated at .710 ($p < .001$).

Behavior

Incidence and types of teaching behavior are presented earlier in this chapter under the heading, "Research Question I."

Correlational Relationships Between the Components A, SN

Attitude and subjective norm are nonsignificantly correlated at .01.

Determinants of Behavioral Intentions

According to Fishbein and Ajzen, behavioral intentions should be predictable from measures of attitude (A) and subjective norm (SN). The appropriate Pearson correlation coefficients for A and SN on behavioral intentions (BI) were calculated. A and SN were regressed on BI. The standardized regression weights provide an estimate of the amount of influence exerted by A and SN as antecedents of BI. The results of these computations are presented in Figure 5.3.

It can be seen that the correlation between A and BI is .80; the correlation between SN and BI is .79. The A beta weight is larger than the SN beta weight. SN and A result in an R value of .82, explaining 67% of the variance between A and SN and BI. The correlation between BI and behavior is very small, less than 1% of the variance is explained by the impact of BI on the behavior.

Table 5.8 presents the product moment correlations between SN, A, BI and the incidence and type of patient teaching. Attitude is significantly correlated with the total number of teaching events and the total number of minutes spent teaching. It is significantly negatively correlated with Type 2 teaching.

Scattergrams constructed for each of the possible relationships failed to indicate any curvilinear relationships. Further polynomial regression was considered unwarranted.

Summary

Attitude and subjective norm contribute to the explanation of the congruence between beliefs and behavioral intentions. The weight of the attitude factor is greater than that of the subjective norm. Correlations between attitude and behavioral intention and between subjective norm and behavioral intention are greater than .7.

There is a low correlation approaching zero between behavioral intention and the behavior specified in the behavioral intentions. There is also

Figure 5.3 Relationships among Attitude, Subjective Norm, Intention
and Behavior

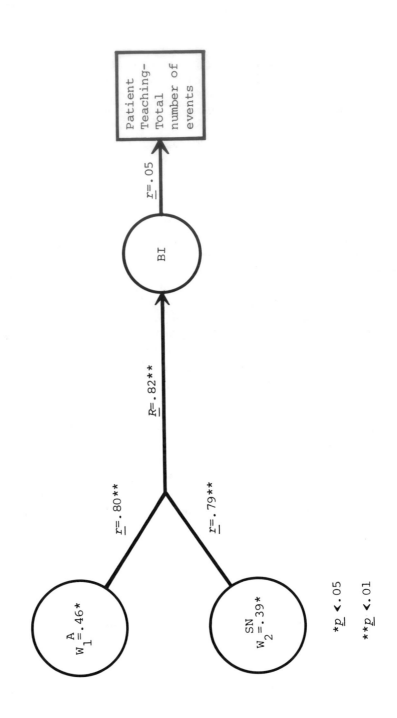

Patient
Teaching-
Total
number of
events

$\underline{r}=.05$

BI

$\underline{R}=.82**$

$\underline{r}=.80**$

$\underline{r}=.79**$

$W_1 \overset{A}{=} .46*$

$W_2 \overset{SN}{=} .39*$

$*\underline{p} <.05$

$**\underline{p} <.01$

Table 5.8. Product Moment Correlations between Components of Fishbein's Behavior Intentions Model and Incidence and Type of Teaching

	A	SN	BI
Total Number Teaching Events	−.54***	.29	.05
Total Minutes Spent Teaching	−.50**	.26	.10
Type 1 Teaching	−.06	.18	.05
Type 2 Teaching	−.63**	.31	.01
Type 3 Teaching	−.04	.10	.12
Type 4 Teaching	−.01	.01	−.08

Note: Two-tailed test of significance
*p < .05
**p < .01
***p < .001

very low correlation between behavioral intentions and the more specific ways in which incidence and type of patient teaching were operationalized. When each component of belief, (A and SN) are correlated with incidence and type of behavior, A is found to be moderately negatively correlated with total number of teaching events, total minutes spent teaching and Type 2 teaching.

Research Question III: What is the Relationship Between the Health Locus of Control Concept and the Behavior Intentions Model?

Table 5.9 presents the correlations between the Multidimensional Health Locus of Control (MHLC) scales and the components of the behavior intentions model. All coefficients approach zero.

Regression of subjective norm and attitude and Multidimensional Health Locus of Control scales on incidence and type of teaching result in multiple R's less than .68, explaining less than 47% of the variance. β weights of PHLC are consistently the highest. The β weights of the other variables are approximately equal. None of the Multiple R's was significant at .05. None of the β weights was significant.

There is almost no correlation between the Multidimensional Health Locus of Control scales and the components (as operationalized) of the behavior intentions model. The use of the MHLC scales and the SN and A as variables in regression on incidence and type of teaching yields low multiple R's and is not likely to be useful in prediction of behavior.

Table 5.9. Product Moment Correlation Between Multidimensional
Health Locus of Control Scales (MHLC) and the Attitude (A),
Subjective Norm (SN) and Behavioral Intentions Model (BIM)

MHLC Scales	A	SN	BIM
PHLC	−.17	−.01	.03
IHLC	−.03	−.10	.01
CHLC	−.14	−.03	.02

General Question: What Factors are Related to the Types and Incidence of Patient Teaching Done by Registered Nurses in the General Hospital?

The first two research questions addressed the major factors this study was designed to explore in relation to incidence and type of patient teaching. This section reports on other variables (such as years of practice, education) which may be related to patient teaching. The basic descriptive statistics have been presented in the sample description.

As demonstrated by Nunnally, phi, point-biserial and rho are only special cases of the product moment correlation formula. The same results are obtained if the product moment formula is used (1967, p. 118). Dichotomous variables are thus reported with continuous variables in Table 5.10 under the product moment heading.

As seen in Table 5.10, holding the baccalaureate degree in nursing as basic education is moderately positively correlated with Types 2 and 4 teaching as well as total number of teaching events and total time spent teaching. Most of the other correlations are low, approaching zero. There is a low negative correlation ($p < .05$) between the number of patients assigned and Type 3 teaching. There is also a low negative correlation between years of practice and Type 1 teaching.

Separate rank order analysis of the favorite facets of nursing activities yielded no relational patterns. Correlational analysis of educational content history with incidence and type of teaching also produced no relational patterns.

Basic nursing education is positively correlated with Types 2 and 4 teaching as well as total number of teaching events and total time spent teaching. Years of nursing practice is negatively correlated with Type 1 teaching. The number of patients assigned is negatively associated with Type 3 teaching. Other factors examined yield correlations approaching zero.

Table 5.10. Product Moment Correlation between Selected Variables and Incidence and Types of Teaching

	Type 1	Type 2	Type 3	Type 4	Total Number Teaching Events	Total Time Spent Teaching
Basic Nursing Education	.19	.40*	.01	.39*	.40*	.52**
Interruptions During Day	-.14	.19	.00	-.05	.10	-.11
Acting as Module Leader	.24	.07	.00	-.18	.05	.00
Medical Unit Assignment	.03	.10	-.24	-.10	-.06	.00
Years of Nursing Practice	-.37*	.02	-.18	-.15	-.13	-.10
Assistant Assigned	-.07	-.16	-.28	.27	-.17	-.09
Number of Patients	-.26	.13	-.34*	.22	-.07	.05

Note Two-tailed test of significance used.
*$p < .05$
**$p < .01$

6

Discussion

Health Locus of Control and
Patient Teaching

Before discussing the relationship between patient teaching and health locus of control it is necessary to examine the reliability of the instruments. The general rule is that a test or scale cannot have a correlation associated with it which is higher than its reliability. The upper limit of the correlation between two variables is the square root of the product of the variables' reliabilities (Asher, 1976). Low reliability thus creates problems in interpreting correlational results. The Multidimensional Health Locus of Control scales' alpha reliabilities ranged from .6 to over .7. The reliability of the observations was measured at the beginning of the study as 99%. The inter-rater reliability for classification of the activities reached 98%. There is, however, the threat that reliability of observation may have slipped despite requests by the observer for occasional reliability checks during observations.

Another area that needs to be examined is the nature of correlational analysis with small numbers of subjects. Nunnally (1967) has written that product moment correlation is often said to have three assumptions that must be met in employing the correlation coefficient: linearity, normal distribution and homoscedasticy. He has pointed out that, unless one of the assumptions were seriously violated, inferential statistics would not be highly in error. With a small number of subjects it becomes somewhat more difficult and important to detect serious violations. One such violation would be correlating a normally distributed variable with scores from a J curve. Via scattergram it was ascertained that no J or curvelinear relationship appeared to exist (although small numbers may be a hindrance in such detection) between variables.

No variable appeared to have a J distribution but not all were normally distributed. As Nunnally (1967) has pointed out, changes in the shape of one distribution tend to have little effect on the magnitude of correlation (less than five points). The results of correlating two continuous variables is thus about the same whether distributions are shaped the same or are somewhat differently shaped. There did not appear to be any obvious heteroscedasticy (spread about the "best fitting" straight line that was different at different levels) although this determination is also hampered somewhat by low numbers. Correlational analysis thus appears provisionally appropriate for detecting presence and direction of relationship between health locus of control and incidence and type of patient teaching.

Incidence of teaching the Teaching Types 1, 2 and 3 are not significantly correlated with any of the Multidimensional Health Locus of Control scales. Chance Health Locus of Control (CHLC) is moderately negatively correlated with teaching about self-care (−.4). Internal Health Locus of Control (IHLC) is moderately positively related to teaching about self-care. These findings could be interpreted to reflect a belief that those who posit control of their health to themselves are also more likely to teach others to care for their own health. Consistent with this interpretation is one that states if there is a belief in chance or fortune as the major controller of health, there is less likelihood of impetus to teach others to care for their own health.

This facile interpretation may be refuted. If the above reasoning is generally true, why then is teaching about positive health practices not positively correlated with IHLC and negatively correlated with CHLC? A strict "Rotter-type" answer might be that the locus of control concept should be used only when there is congruence between the behavior and the locus of control measure. In this case it would be patient teaching locus of control. Theoretically one might expect no correlation.

A better interpretation may rest somewhere between the two positions. Health care personnel's clinical behavior is popularly believed to be somewhat related to personal beliefs. Examples of such behavior include advice given about smoking, child rearing, resuscitation efforts. This, however, is not a perfect relationship and is affected by professional education and years of practice. In the case at hand a multifactorial analysis is not possible due to small cell size. Future study may show differential impacts on patient teaching. The combination of education and practice experience may be a more powerful attenuator of the relationship of health locus on teaching about self-care. The problem obviously requires more study. If researchers of the future are not interested in the possible relationship of personal health locus of control and teaching but rather the relationship of the nurse's estimate of the patient's health locus of control and teaching, new scales will have to be developed.

From the results, it does not appear that health locus of control significantly contributes to understanding the factors which may influence patient teaching. If future studies confirm that there is no relationship, this may be beneficial to the efforts to increase patient teaching. The challenge of designing programs to alter health locus of control in a group whose professional life is devoted to health care would be tremendous. Beliefs are often among the most expensive and difficult variables to influence.

Beliefs, Attitudes, Intentions and Behaviors

The discussion of reliability and correlational analysis in health locus of control and patient teaching also applies to the results for beliefs, attitudes, intentions and behaviors. The alpha reliabilities for attitude (A) and subjective norm (SN) were above .7.

The predictors of the behavioral intention (BI)— attitude and subjective norm—are consistent with other reported work. Correlations between attitude and behavioral intention and subejctive norm and behavioral intention are all greater than .79. The R is high and significant, $R = .82, p < .01$. The weight of attitude is greater than that of subjective norm. This finding is supported by previous research (Ajzen and Fishbein, 1980). Behavioral intention is not appreciably correlated with patient teaching incidence or type.

It is interesting to note that R was not measurably increased by the addition of subjective norm to the equation already containing attitude. The reason for this is not clear although there may be some computational artifact due to the already high correlations of attitude and subjective norm with behavioral intention.

Fishbein and Ajzen (1975) have cited several reasons why there may not be accurate prediction of behavior from stated behavior. These factors include length of time between statement of intention and performance of the behavior, the sequence of events necessary to perform the behavior, dependence on others' help, habit and lack of ability.

In 1980, these authors wrote that intentions should always predict behavior providing the measure of intention corresponds to the behavioral criteria and the intention does not change prior to performance (p. 50). The other factors moderate the intention-behavior relationship only if the second condition is not met. A strong intention-behavior relationship will be obtained if intention is measured after the extraneous factors occur. They further suggest using appropriate behavioral anchors in eliciting intentions and measuring behaviors. As previously worded, some items may represent behavioral categories (sets of actions) rather than single behaviors. Unfortunately, this further delineation of behavior was published after data collection for this study was complete. This deviation in wording from the latest formulation could account for some of the lack of behavior-intention correlation.

Nurses may have exhibited incongruence between intention and behavior because there was no perceived need to perform the behavior. This argument is to be challenged on the basis of the observations. Several times patients asked the observer to explain things to them. There were also many situations where the observer noted missed teaching opportunities.

Another reason for incongruence may be a contamination of behavioral intention and attitude by ethical desirability. There was almost no variance in the behavioral intention to teach nor was there in attitude toward teaching. Professional socialization may have made it almost impossible for nurses to rate these two items any other way than "strongly probable/possible." Considering the now apparent specificity problem referred to above, this may account for quite a bit of incongruence.

Although intention was not remeasured after what Fishbein and Ajzen are now calling moderating variables may have interfered, it may be helpful to consider these variables. Interruptions were not negatively correlated (or correlated at all) with incidence and types of teaching. Exposure to a course does not admittedly guarantee skill; however, all nurses reported exposure in some way to content on patient teaching so that the explanation of a total lack of skill appears unlikely. Exposure to such courses was not correlated with patient teaching.

HLC and Beliefs, Attitudes, Intentions and Behaviors

There is no correlation between health locus of control and attitude, perceived subjective norm and behavioral intention. It thus appears there is no relationship between health locus of control and even the intention to teach and no relationship between attitude and health locus of control. As described above this may be a spurious conclusion because of the possible measurement problems associated with attitude and behavioral intention. Due to the strong possibility of social desirability/ethical influence on attitude and behavioral intention, it is not possible to discuss accurately the meaning of the finding of no relationship.

General Considerations Related to Patient Teaching

The health locus of control concept does not appear especially useful in the context of patient teaching. The Fishbein model may be helpful in predicting intention but not in discussing actual teaching behavior. Popular wisdom might suggest other factors, some of which were incidentally measured by this study. These factors include education, discontinuity as measured by interruptions, shift in role as in acting as charge nurse, experience as measured by years of practice and work load as measured by number of patients and helpers.

Basic educational preparation is moderately positively correlated with total number of teaching events (.4), time spent teaching (.52), teaching about current disease states and teaching for home self-care. Content experiences in various aspects of patient teaching were not so correlated. There may be an element of skill or habit or prioritizing in baccalaureate education that accounts for this difference.

Interruptions, acting as charge nurse and unit assignment were factors not significantly related to incidence or type of teaching. Years of nursing practice was moderately negatively correlated (-.37) with teaching about hospital procedures and rules. It was not correlated with any other aspect of teaching. One could argue the more familiar one is with routine the less likely one is to explain it to others.

Having an assistant appears to have no significant relation to patient teaching. In a primary care situation, if patient assignments are equitable, this would be expected. The nurse would still be with the patient the same amount of time in her role as a professional, the assistant being assigned to more of the nonpatient contact situations (getting water pitchers ready, disposing of linen, making beds). The number of patients also does not appear to be generally significantly related to patient teaching. There must, of course, be a limit to the number of patients for whom the nurse, regardless of the nonprofessional help assigned, can continue to provide care without there being a negative relationship with patient teaching. The increase in the amount of paperwork alone would decrease time available for teaching.

Beyond discussion of these factors and their relation to patient teaching, it is also important to discuss this study's observations of patient teaching. The average of 4.9 teaching events per nurse indicates that not every patient received teaching. Further, some patients had more than one teaching session.

The average number of minutes per event is a low 3.78 with a standard deviation of 2.04. The longest period was nine minutes. It appears that most of the teaching is incidental rather than planned. The average total number of minutes spent teaching as 17.6 This too does not appear to be a large amount of time. Taken as a percentage of total time, this average is more noteworthy. Teaching accounted on average for eight percent of the observation period, a surprise to the observer since during observation it did not appear that this much teaching was occurring. This perception was shared by the subjects who would often informally apologize for "not teaching at all." The figures indicated otherwise.

To put this study in proper perspective it is also necessary to discuss the teaching types. These labels for content were comparatively easy for the rater to apply reliably. They also were reported to have high face validity by nurse experts. It was anticipated that there would be occasional situations in which there would be a content-type mix. In only six situations did this occur. The short time for any one teaching event may account for this finding.

That teaching about current disease pathology and treatment is almost three times more likely than any other type of teaching is possibly explained by the situation in which most hospital patients find themselves. The ethical, legal and professional priority of the nurse is to teach about the disease and its treatment so that the patient can give informed consent and in some cases, so that anxiety about the unknown can be alleviated.

This need to prioritize was evident to the observer. The nurses were subjected to almost continual interruptions that could not be postponed. In anticipation of this, the nurses would begin certain tasks early in the observation period that they knew would be priorities later in the shift (example, medication preparation). The nurses often phrased this as "things that have to be done before the day gets crazy." Patient teaching is not easily or appropriately done at 0730; thus even if patient teaching is a priority it is relegated to the later morning hours when there are still more competing priorities. This perhaps lessens the incidence of teaching. A re-analysis of times when most interruptions occur instead of total interruptions might be helpful in the future.

Finally, some comments on the effect of the nonparticipant observer may help in the interpretation of the findings. Clinical investigation requires the enlistment of subjects. As the topic involved an area of professional practice, subjects were understandably reticent but, once a nurse on a unit had taken part in the study, this reticence evaporated.

Remaining a nonparticipant observer was a problem not so easily solved. In one case the observer noted an incorrect dosage of parenteral medication had been calculated. This required intervention. Other incidents occurred in which the nurses included the observer in the situation. For example, one nurse was doing discharge teaching with a cancer patient. She told the patient that the observer had had experience in this area and suggested the patient talk with the researcher about the illness. At other times patients directly asked the observer questions about their conditions or requested assistance. In these cases patients were referred to their nurse.

Although it is not possible to assess accurately the effect of the nonparticipant observer, some impressions may be helpful. The nurses were so busy in most instances that any effect was probably attenuated somewhat. The nurses' activities often required such concentration that anything not necessary to the activity was ignored. The nurses had also recently had experience with being observed due to various quality care audits, pharmacy programs and orientation programs. This may also have helped decrease the effect of the observer. One other factor also supports this idea. Nurses in the study estimated their amount of teaching the same as they did in the pilot when no observation was made. It appears they did not artificially increase the amount of patient teaching when under observation.

7

Conclusions and Implications

The data from this study indicate that there is wide variation in the incidence of patient teaching by registered nurses and that there is some variation in the content taught. It appears that health locus of control is not strongly related to these behaviors. It also appears that despite nurses' (1) belief in the importance of regularly including patient teaching as a part of nursing care, (2) having generally positive attitudes toward patient teaching and (3) perceiving that referents expect them to teach, nurses' behavior does not directly correspond with their behavioral intentions to teach. Attitude and perceived expectation do, however, clearly influence behavioral intentions.

The difference between behavioral intentions and behavior does not appear to be related to interruption, number of patients assigned or presence of an assistant. Using health locus of control in combination with behavioral intention also does not increase the correlation with observed teaching behavior.

Original nursing education shows some positive relationship with incidence of teaching and in teaching certain content about disease processes and self-care at home.

The results of this study contribute to the limited body of knowledge regarding actual incidence of patient teaching. It appears nurses underestimate the amount they do teach and do not accurately report in retrospect the kind of teaching they do. Nurses appear to be concerned about evaluating their performance in this area. After being observed they often asked for their clinical practices to be evaluated and for suggestions. Nurses also seem to be bombarded by multiple task demands and frequent interruptions. The requests for evaluation in such a situation indicate a sincere desire to provide quality patient teaching.

The results also contribute to the body of knowledge regarding the application of the Fishbein model of intentional behavior. The model was useful in predicting behavioral intentions but not in predicting behavior. The model may need reformulation in order to account for the multiple variables which exist in any social behavior situation, abstract values and possible unintentional contamination of what the model defines as attitude by desirability factors.

Finally, although the results do not appear to indicate a strong relationship between health locus of control and patient teaching behavior, the study does contribute to the continuing fund of knowledge about the Multidimensional Health Locus of Control scales. The subjects' scores were highly consistent with those previously reported for professional women. All scales continued to indicate high internal consistency.

Implications for Practice, Administration and Education

This study has implications for nursing practice and nursing administration. Practicing nurses may need to reexamine their perceptions of patient teaching. Many of the nurses who insisted they had done little or no teaching were among the highest incidence teachers. Nurses need to be conscious of the fact that they often teach in other than the traditional seated teaching session. Nurses do not appear to credit themselves for what they do. Considering the heavy responsibilities of patient counseling, performance of pychomotor tasks and the management of other members of the health team, staff nurses who spend 7% of the busy morning period in patient teaching are to be commended.

Another reason nurses may underestimate their teaching is their perception of their skill (or lack of skill) in teaching. As noted, all subjects reportedly had received education in assessment of learning needs. When they did not do what they felt was a complete assessment or perhaps did not have time to complete a written plan, they may have thought of themselves as not teaching at all. A more systematic evaluation of personal practice may be indicated.

This evaluation of practice might be aided by the four types of teaching as defined in this study. The types are easy to understand and apparently wide enough in scope to cover the kinds of teaching done by staff nurses. A reexamination of the perception of what activities constitute patient teaching may also be helpful. It is possible that only time spent in patient contact is perceived as teaching and that planning activities or evaluation activities are not included.

Nursing administrators should also note the discrepancy between nurses' reports and their observed behavior. Many institutions are hiring auditors for patient care studies. Self-report on written forms is a frequent method of data gathering although in some studies non-nurse observers are used. It is possible patient teaching is under reported. The nurse may place on the form a check indicating preparation for x-ray study. In reality the nurse may not only have physically prepared the patient for a barium study but may also have taught the patient about some positive health practices.

The profession has long used the term "incidental" or "informal" teaching. The frequency of this teaching and its impact are not measured by the data gathering mechanisms popular today. These data may lead to inappropriate decisions that nurses need not be the caregivers in certain situations.

The finding that there is considerable informal teaching occurring even during the busy morning hours of nursing care should not be construed as totally comforting. Research has shown "formal" teaching to be more effective than "informal" teaching especially when multiple behaviors are to be learned (Millazzo, 1980). If nursing management has made a commitment to patient education, systems must be devised so that administrators have specific information on the macrolevel in terms of patient education needs. The typology used in this study might prove helpful in making these judgments. For example, more Type 3 teaching may be needed in one hospital than another. Nursing managers need to be able to quantify these needs to appropriately secure and distribute resources, i.e. nurses prepared to teach both formally and informally.

This study raises some questions about these resources. The study suggests that there is a positive relationship between baccalaureate education and the total incidence of teaching and some teaching types. If, through further study, this relationship between patient teaching and nursing education can be confirmed, there are great implications for assignment priorities and desirable employment mix.

Nursing educators may be most interested in exploring the reason for this finding. According to one line of reasoning, the baccalaureate prepared nurses have probably had more exposure to teaching/learning principles and methods and should, therefore, be more comfortable in teaching. They would thus be more likely to teach. A counter argument might be that the baccalaureate nurses have been more sensitized or socialized into this aspect of the nursing role. It must be remembered that this study is descriptive in nature and by its design and purpose unsuited to establishing cause and effect. Another study would be necessary to support either of these rationales.

The finding of no relationship between interruptions, number of patients assigned and the number of assistants and incidence and type of teaching should also be viewed with caution. As described in the Chapter 6, there are several reasons this finding might be spurious. The results cannot be seen as an endorsement for increasing interruptions or work load even if these findings are confirmed. This study made no attempt to determine if all patient learning needs were being met. It is possible that even those nurses who ranked as high incidence teachers but who had many interruptions and extra duties did not meet all patient learning needs. The brief time spent per incident and the incident per patient ratio support this contention.

Finally, nursing practice and administration might consider the behavior intentions model when analyzing patient education activities. It appears that strongly favorable attitudes and powerful subjective norm components explain the strength of intention to teach in general. It also appears that various factors may make it impossible to carry out the behavioral intention.

A first step to analysis would be to ascertain to what extent teaching behaviors adhere to the institution's standards. If behaviors meet the standards, no further investigation may be necessary. If behaviors are found inadequate, practitioner intentions can be measured using the relatively simple methods outlined by the model. If intentions are found to be high, the support system may need to be redesigned. This redesign may include assisting with improvement of teaching abilities, provision of a different mechanism for distribution of teaching aids, reassignment of duties that lead to priority conflicts or the addition of personnel. If intentions are found to be low, the attitudes and subjective norms can be measured. Strategies can then be devised to begin to affect these areas. For example, after determination of the significant others influencing the subjective norm, appropriate steps can be taken to influence the impact these people have on the nurse in relation to patient teaching.

Implications for Research

The results of this study have many implications for future research. These implications include the following areas: design, data analysis, instrumentation and conceptual formulations.

Design

Future studies which measure teaching should consider employing direct observation, not retrospective self-report. As the differences between the pilot study and the actual research indicate, self-report is widely variant from actual practice.

An increase in the number of subjects would permit the use of alternate statistical methods, resulting in greater confidence in interpretation of results as well as an increased ability to study specific aspects of the problem. Acquiring subjects in nursing research is costly in terms of time and resources. As a result, much of nursing research suffers from the same problem, i.e. inadequate numbers. Future researchers should place great emphasis on enlisting adequate resources for full measure to be received from efforts expended.

The use of more than one institution would further increase generalizability. Using numerous institutions would have the secondary benefit of enabling study of one more potential variable in incidence of patient teaching, that is, the nursing care delivery system. A comparison of primary nursing, functional nursing, and team nursing may lead to interesting data that could explain differences in teaching practices. In this study, despite the policy of using a primary/modular approach, some differences in delivery systems appeared to be present from floor to floor. With greater numbers and a more pronounced variance in delivery system, delivery systems' relationships to teaching practices might be determined.

Data Analysis

Transcripts of observations may provide a source of data that may assist in analyzing related questions. One of these questions deals with the relationship of personal health locus of control and the locus of control orientation of common with patients. Is there an identifiable locus of control bias in nurses' statements to patients? Is that bias congruent with the nurses' health locus of control? If there is an identifiable pattern, another study could be designed to assess change in the patients' locus of control over time as a result of exposure to a health care worker. What effect does change in health locus of control have on patients' health practices?

Future analysis of the role identification data might also identify factors related to nurses' behavior and patient teaching. There may be a relationship between role perception and behavior that is not evident in relationships between either the health locus of control or behavior intentions model and behavior. This possibility is discussed in more detail in the section on conceptual formulations.

Instrumentation

Confidence in a study's results can only be as strong as confidence in the instruments. In future work, better ways to record nursing behavior and qualify the results might be attempted. Use of standard situations for nurse subjects to respond to might be employed. Such developments require research projects in and of themselves. If such instruments could be designed, some of the reliability concerns expressed in the Chapter 6 would be relieved.

Another area for future research includes the exploration of alternate ways to measure the components of the behavior intentions model. After the present study was planned and data collected, Ajzen and Fishbein (1980) described alternate ways to measure components of the model including alternate ways to measure behavior. Their Index of Behavioral Categories may be useful to subsequent workers as an alternate instrument for measuring the behavior intentions model's components. Social behavior is difficult to predict due to its multivariable complexity. As the results of this study indicate, if the behavior intentions model is to prove useful in application to these situations, improvement in definition is necessary.

Conceptual Formulations

It appears that the health locus of control and the components of the behavior intentions model may not be powerfully related to incidence and type of teaching. Several alternatives might exist in the search for a conceptual framework on which to base future research.

The first possibility is to investigate the contribution role theory may make. This is a promising area of research if the possibility of social desirability can be eliminated or at least controlled. As discussed in Chapter 6, it is open to debate whether obtained attitude and behavioral intention components of this study were tainted by social desirability. Unless carefully constructed, role studies might have the same problem.

Another alternative is to approach the general question using a more traditional Rotter-like approach to locus of control. In the strict construction of this theory, locus of control of patient teaching would be measured, not health locus of control. An appropriate teaching locus of control instrument would, of course, need to be constructed.

A third possibility is to reexamine the question in light of Fishbein and Ajzen's newest work (1980). In several ways this work differs from the earlier (1975) volume. There is an unresolved problem that part of the subjective norm should be measured with either general desire to comply statements *or* behavior specific desire to comply statements. There is also greater emphasis on the use of the theory to measure general behaviors. Beyond examining the question using Fishbein and Ajzen's theory of reasoned action (as they now refer to it), future research might also find it useful to incorporate Jaccard's (1976) concept of moral obligation. In nursing there are many demands. The nurse may intend to teach but her sense of moral obligation to give pain medication may be greater than her sense of obligation to teach. Similarly, Triandis's suggestion (1977) that a separate measure of perceived consequences of performing a behavior as well as a measure of attitude be used might also be useful. This separate measure may also avoid some of the social desirability problems mentioned in Chapter 6. Research concerning the construct validity of belief, attitude and intention should also be continued. If beliefs and attitudes are so highly correlated with intention, are they parts of a larger construct? Is it useful to measure attitudes if the same results are obtained via behavioral intention measurement? Many questions remain to be answered.

Appendix A

Nurse Questionnaire

There are many factors which affect the nurse's relationship with the patient. The purpose of this section of the questionnaire is to describe yourself as a teacher of patients.

Rate the meaning of the phrase presented below on the series of adjective scales beneath it. If you feel that the phrase is very closely related to the word at one end of the scale, you should place an X in a space close to the word:

Example
exciting __:__:__:__:__:__: X dull

If you feel the phrase is only slightly related to one side as opposed to the other, you should put your X closer to the center:

Example
humorous __:__: X :__:__:__:__ serious

It is important that you place your X only in a space, that you place only one X on each line and that you check every scale. Make each item a separate and independent judgment. Work at a high speed through these scales - do not puzzle over individual items. It is your first impression - your immediate feelings - that are wanted.

MYSELF, A TEACHER OF PATIENTS

passive	__:__:__:__:__:__	active
unimportant	__:__:__:__:__:__	important
calm	__:__:__:__:__:__	excitable
optimistic	__:__:__:__:__:__	pessimistic
submissive	__:__:__:__:__:__	dominant
bad	__:__:__:__:__:__	good

MYSELF, A TEACHER OF PATIENTS

structured	__:__:__:__:__:__	unstructured
heavy	__:__:__:__:__:__	light
successful	__:__:__:__:__:__	unsuccessful
relaxed	__:__:__:__:__:__	tense
sad	__:__:__:__:__:__	happy
constrained	__:__:__:__:__:__	free
slow	__:__:__:__:__:__	fast
strong	__:__:__:__:__:__	weak
fair	__:__:__:__:__:__	unfair
dynamic	__:__:__:__:__:__	static

Another factor affecting the nurse's relationship with patients includes his/her belief system and the other demands of the nurse's job. Please indicate with a circle your answers to the questions below.

	Extremely Improbable or Unimportant						Extremely Probable or Important
1. How important is it to routinely include patient teaching during nursing care?	1	2	3	4	5	6	7
2. How probable is it that you routinely include patient teaching in your nursing care?	1	2	3	4	5	6	7

Now, please rate the behavior described below on the four adjective scales. Place an X at any point along the scale to indicate the extent to which the behavior is best described by one or the other of the two adjectives in each scale. Use only one X on each scale and check each scale - do not omit any.

BEHAVIOR: Routinely including patient teaching
            as a part of nursing care.

foolish   __:__:__:__:__:__ wise

good   __:__:__:__:__:__ bad

harmful   __:__:__:__:__:__ beneficial

rewarding   __:__:__:__:__:__ punishing

The next section asks about your general beliefs
regarding health and illness. Each statement is a
belief statement with which you may agree or disagree.
For each item, circle on the scale how you feel.   One (1)
means you strongly disagree and six (6) means you
strongly agree. The more strongly you agree with the
statements, the higher the number you will pick. The
more strongly you disagree, the lower the number will
be. Since this is a measure of your beliefs, there are
no right or wrong answers.

As much as you can, try to answer each item
independently. Try not to be influenced by your previous
choices. Work quickly. It is important that you
respond according to your actual beliefs and not
according to how you feel you should believe or how you
think anyone wants you to believe. (Please turn the page
and begin.)

		Strongly Disagree	Moderately Disagree	Slightly Disagree	Slightly Agree	Moderately Agree	Strongly Agree
1.	If I get sick, it is my own behavior which determines how soon I get well again.	1	2	3	4	5	6
2.	No matter what I do, if I am going to get sick, I will get sick.	1	2	3	4	5	6
3.	Having regular contact with my physician is the best way for me to avoid illness.	1	2	3	4	5	6
4.	Most things that affect my health happen to me by accident.	1	2	3	4	5	6
5.	Whenever I don't feel well, I should consult a medically trained professional.	1	2	3	4	5	6
6.	I am in control of my health.	1	2	3	4	5	6
7.	My family has a lot to do with my becoming sick or staying well.	1	2	3	4	5	6
8.	When I get sick I am to blame.	1	2	3	4	5	6
9.	Luck plays a big part in determining how soon I will recover from an illness.	1	2	3	4	5	6
10.	Health professionals control my health.	1	2	3	4	5	6
11.	My good health is largely a matter of good fortune.	1	2	3	4	5	6
12.	The main thing which affects my health is what I myself do.	1	2	3	4	5	6

	Strongly Disagree	Moderately Disagree	Slightly Disagree	Slightly Agree	Moderately Agree	Strongly Agree
13. If I take care of myself, I can avoid illness.	1	2	3	4	5	6
14. When I recover from an illness, it's usually because other people (for example, doctors, nurses, family friends) have been taking good care of me.	1	2	3	4	5	6
15. No matter what I do, I'm likely to get sick.	1	2	3	4	5	6
16. If it's meant to be, I will stay healthy.	1	2	3	4	5	6
17. If I take the right actions, I can stay healthy.	1	2	3	4	5	6
18. Regarding my health, I can only do what my doctor tells me to do.	1	2	3	4	5	6

The nurse's relation ship with patients also depends in part on his/her perception of the expectations of other people and desire to comply with those expectations. Please indicate with a circle how probable the following statements are. One is extremely improbable and seven is extremely probable.

	Extremely Improbable						Extremely Probable
1. My head nurse thinks I should routinely include patient teaching in my care.	1	2	3	4	5	6	7
1a. I want to comply with what my head nurse thinks about including patient teaching.	1	2	3	4	5	6	7

	Extremely Improbable					Extremely Probable	

2. Nurses on this unit think
    I should routinely include
    patient teaching in my care. 1   2   3   4   5   6   7

2a. I want to comply with what
    nurses on this unit think
    about including patient
    teaching.   1   2   3   4   5   6   7

3. Most of my patients think I
    should routinely include
    patient teaching in my care. 1   2   3   4   5   6   7

3a. I want to comply with what
    my patients think about in-
    cluding patient teaching.   1   2   3   4   5   6   7

4. The majority of members of my
    profession think I should
    routinely include patient
    teaching in my care.   1   2   3   4   5   6   7

4a. I want to comply with what
    the majority of member of
    my profession think about in-
    cluding patient teaching.   1   2   3   4   5   6   7

5. Attending physicians think I
    should routinely include pa-
    tient teaching in my care.   1   2   3   4   5   6   7

5a. I want to comply with what the
    attending physicians think about
    including patient teaching. 1   2   3   4   5   6   7

Finally, please rate the behavior described below as you
think other nurses on your unit would rate it.

BEHAVIOR: Routinely including patient teaching in nursing
           care.

              foolish   __:__:__:__:__:__:__   wise
                 good   __:__:__:__:__:__:__   bad
              harmful   __:__:__:__:__:__:__   beneficial
             rewarding   __:__:__:__:__:__:__   punishing

DEMOGRAPHIC INFORMATION

Please circle one answer for each question below unless otherwise instructed.

1. Please indicate <u>all</u> degrees you hold and the year you graduated.

   a. __diploma in nursing__year   e. __MA/MS__year
   b. __AA/AD__year   f. __MSN__year
   c. __BA/BS__year   g. __other(specify)
   d. __BSN__year

   If you hold MSN, please indicate clinical specialty._____

2. What is the approximate number of years of your clinical practice of nursing?_____

3. What is the approximate number of years in positions where patient teaching is to be expected?_____

4. Your current position title is _____.
   Your type of unit is chiefly:
       a. medical
       b. surgical
       c. other (specify)_____

5. How long have you been at this position?_____

6. Your employment is:
       a. full time
       b. part time (specify)_____

7. How long have you been at this hospital?_____

8. How would you rank the importance - in terms of <u>interest</u> <u>to</u> <u>you</u> - the following facets of nursing activities? Please cross out any activities which do not apply to your job and then rank from 1 (one), most important, to 5 or 6, least important.

   ____performing skilled procedures
   ____coordinating and teaching other health care
        team members
   ____patient advocacy (representing patient interests
        to others)
   ____patient teaching
   ____patient observation and recording
   ____other (specify)

9. Circle the content areas your educational experiences
    have included and indicate with a check where these
    experiences took place.

	Under Graduate	MSN Graduate	Cont. Education
a. assessment of patient learning needs			
b. use and selection of audio/visual aids			
c. classroom and group teaching methods			
d. strategies to increase patient compliance with teaching suggestions			

Appendix B

Observer Recording Form

Subject No. :

No. of Patients :

Assistants :

Extra Duties :

Intent to Teach :

Comments :

Time	Activity	Initiator	Participants	Notes

Bibliography

Ajzen I., Fishbein M.: Attitudinal and normative variables as predictors of specific behaviors. *J Pers Soc Psych* 27:47-57, 1973.

———: Attitude-behavior relations: A theoretical analysis and review of empirical research. *Psych Bull* 84:888-918, 1977.

———: *Understanding Attitudes and Predicting Social Behavior.* Englewood Cliffs, New Jersey: Prentice Hall, 1980.

Anderson L. R., Fishbein M.: Prediction of attitude from the number, strength and evaluative aspects of beliefs about the attitude object: A comparison of summation and congruity theories. *J Pers and Soc Psychol* 3:437-443, 1965.

Asher J. W.: *Educational Research and Evaluation Methods.* Boston: Little, Brown and Company, 1976.

Balch P., Ross A. W.: Predicting success in weight reduction as a function of locus of control. A unidimensional and multidimensional approach. *J Consult Clin Psychol* 43:119, 1975.

Bauman D. E., Udry J. R.: Powerlessness and regularity of contraception in an urban Negro male sample: A research note. *J Marr Fam* 34:112-114, 1972.

Bentler P. M., Speckart G.: Models of attitude-behavior relations. *Psych Rev* 86:452-464, 1979.

Berkowitz N. H., Malone M. F., Klein M. W., Eaton A.: Patient follow-through in the outpatient department. *Nurs Res* 12:16-22, 1963.

Best J. A.: Tailoring smoking withdrawal procedures to personality and motivational differences. *J Consult Clin Psychol* 43:1-8, 1975.

Best J. S., Steffy R. A.: Smoking modification tailored to subject characteristics. *Behav Ther* 2:177-191, 1971.

Blue Cross Association: White Paper: Patient health education. Chicago, The Association, 1974.

Carlson A. R.: The relationship between behavioral intention, attitude toward the behavior and normative beliefs about the behavior. Doctoral dissertation: U of Illinois, 1968.

Cohen S. A., Mazzuca S. A., Vinicor F., Clark C. M.: Physicians' beliefs as predictors of their clinical intentions. A paper presented at the annual meeting of the AERA, Boston, April 1980.

Cohen S. A.: Patient education: a review of the literature. *J of Adv Nursing* 6:11-18, 1981.

Cromwell R. L. Butterfield E. C., Brayfield P. M., Curry J. J.: *Acute Myocardial Infarction: Reaction and Recovery.* St. Louis, C. V. Mosby, 1977.

Dabbs J. M., Kirscht J. P.: "Internal control" and the taking of influenza shots. *Psychol Rep* 28:959-962, 1971.

Darrow W. W.: Innovative health behavior: A study of the use, acceptance and use-effectiveness of the condom as a venereal disease prophylactic. *Diss Abstr Int* 34A:2792A, 1973.

Davidson A. R., Jacard J.. J.: Variables that moderate the attitude behavior relation: Results of a longitudinal survey. *J Pers Soc Psych* 37:1364-1376, 1979.

Fisch M. A.: Internal versus external ego orientation and family planning effectiveness among poor black women. *Diss Abstr Int* 35 (2B):1045-1046, 1974.

Fishbein M.: An investigation of the relationships between beliefs about an object and the attitude toward that object. *Human Rel* 16:233-39, 1963.

————: A consideration of beliefs and their role in attitude measurement. In Fishbein M. (ed): *Readings in Attitude, Theory and Measurement.* New York, J. Wiley and Sons Inc., 1967.

————: Attitude and the prediction of behavior. In Fishbein M. (ed): *Readings in Attitude, Theory and Measurement.* New York, J. Wiley and Sons Inc., 1967.

Fishbein M., Ajzen I.: Attitudes towards objects as predictors of single and multiple behavioral criteria. *Psych Rev* 81:59-74, 1974.

————: *Belief, Attitude, Intention and Behavior.* Reading, Massachusetts, Addison-Wesley, 1975.

————: On construct validity: A critique of Miniard and Cohen's paper. *J Exper Soc Psychol* 17:340-350, 1981.

Fishbein M., Coombs F. S.: Basis for decision: An attitudinal analysis of voting behavior. *J Appl Soc Psychol* 4:95-124, 1974.

Fishbein M., Hunter R.: Summation versus balance in attitude organization and change. *J Abnorm Soc Psych* 69:505-510, 1964.

Fishbein M., Raven B. H.: The AB scales: An operational definition of belief and attitude. *Human Rel* 15:35-44, 1962.

Freidson E.: Dominant professions, bureaucracy, and client services. In Rosengren W. R., Lefton M.: *Organizations and Clients; Essays in the Sociology of Service.* Columbus, Ohio, Charles Merrill Publishing Company, 1970.

Golladay F.: U. S. National Center for Health Services Research and Development, Economic Analysis Branch. Rockville, Maryland, The Center, 1973.

Gough H. G.: A factor analysis of contraceptive preferences. *J Psychol* 84:199-210, 1973.

Grotelueschen A. D., Caulley D. N.: A rationale for studying determinants on intention to participate in continuing professional education. Occasional Paper, Office for Study of Continuing Professional Education, U of Illinois at Urbana-Champaign #3, 1977.

Huck S. W., Cormier W. H., Bound W. G.: *Reading statistics and research.* New York, Harper and Row, 1974.

Jaccard J. J., Davidson A. R.: Toward and understanding of family planning behaviors. An initial investigation. *J Appl Soc Psych* 2:228-235, 1972.

Jaccard J., King G. W.: A probabilistic model of the relationship between beliefs and behavioral intentions. *Human Commun Res* 3:332-342, 1977.

Jaccard J., Knox R., Brinberg D.: Prediction of behavior from beliefs: An extension and test of a subjective probability model. *J Pers Soc Psych* 37:1239-1248, 1979.

James W. H., Woodruff A. B., Werner W.: Effect in internal and external control upon changes in smoking behavior. *J Consut Psychol* 29:184-186, 1965.

Jeffery D. B., Christensen E. R.: The relative efficacy of behavior therapy, will power and no-treatment control procedures for weight loss. Paper presented at the Association for Advancement of Behavior Therapy, New York, 1972.

Joe V.C.: Review of the internal-external control construct as a personality variable. *Psychol Rep* 28:619-640, 1971.

Johnson J. E., Dabbs J. M., Leventhal H.: Psychosocial factors in the welfare of surgical patients. *Nurs Res:* 17-18-19, 1970.

Keller A. B., Simms J. H., Herry W. E., et al.: Psychological sources of "resistance to family planning." *Merrill-Palmer Quarterly* 16:286-302, 1970.

Kirscht, J. P.: Perceptions of control and health beliefs. *Can J Behav Sci* 4:225-237, 1972.

Lee E. A., Garvey J. L.: How is inpatient education being managed? *Nurs Dig* 6:1, 12-16, 1978.

Levenson H.: Activism and powerful others: Distinctions within the concept of internal-external control. *J Pers Assess* 38:377-383, 1974.

————: Multidimensional locus of control in psychiatric patients. *J Consul Clin Psychol* 41:397-404, 1973.

Lichtenstein E., Kreutzer C. S.: Further normative and correlation data on internal-external (I—E) control of reinforcement scale. *Psychol Rep* 21:1014-1016, 1967.

Lowery B. W.: Disease-related learning and disease- control in diabetics as a function of locus of control. *Diss Abstr Int* 35 (6-A):352B, 1974.

Lowery B. W., DuCette J. P.: Disease-related and disease-control in diabetics as a function of locus of control. *Nurs Res* 25:358-362, 1976.

MacDonald A. P. Jr: Internal-external locus of control and the practice of birth control. *Psychol Rep* 27:206, 1970.

————: Internal-external locus of control. In Robinson J. P., Shaver P. (eds): *Measures of Social Psychological Attitudes.* Ann Arbor, Institute for Social Research, University of Michigan, 1973.

Malone M., Berkowitz N. H., Klein M. W.: Interpersonal conflict in the outpatient department. *Am J Nurs* 62:108-112, 1962.

Manno B., Marston A. R.: Weight reduction as a function of negative covert reinforcement (sensitization) versus positive covert reinforcement. *Behav Res Ther* 10:201-207, 1972.

McArdle J. B.: Positive and negative communications and subsequent attitude and behavior change in alcoholics. Doctoral dissertation: U of Illinois, 1972.

McCulloch C., Boggs B., Varner C.: Implementation of educational programs for patients *Nurs admin Q* 4:61-65, 1980.

Millazzo V.: A study of the difference in health knowledge gained through formal and informal teaching. *Heart and Lung* 9:1079-1082, 1980.

Miniard P., Cohen J. B.: An examination of the Fishbein Ajzen behavioral intentions model's concepts and measures. *J Exper Soc Psychol* 17:309-339, 1981.

Moses E., Roth A.: Nursepower. *Am J Nurs* 79:1745-1756, 1979.

Murdaugh C.L.: Effects of nurses' knowledge of teaching-learning principles on knowledge of coronary care unit patients. *Heart and Lung* 1073-1078, 1980.

Nunnally J.: *Psychometric Theory.* New York, McGraw Hill, 1967.

O'Bryan G. G.: The relationship between an individual's I—E orientation and information seeking, learning and use of weight control relevant information. *Diss Abstr Int* 33B:447B, 1972.

Palm M.: Recognizing opportunities for informal patient teaching. *Nurs Clinics* 6:669-678, 1978.

Parcel G. S., Mayer M. P.: Development of an instrument to measure children's health locus of control. *Health Ed Monogr* 6:149-159, 1978.

Phares E. J.: *Locus of Control in Personality.* Morristown, New Jersey, General Learning Press, 1976.

Pohl M. L.: Teaching activities of the nursing practitioner. *Nurs Res* 14:4-11, 1965.

Redman B.: *The Process of Patient Teaching in Nursing.* St. Louis, C. V. Mosby Company, 1976.

————: Patient education in hospitals: Developmental issues. *J Nurs Admin* 8:28-30, 1981.

————(ed): *Patterns for Distribution of Patient Education.* New York, Appleton-Century-Crofts, 1981.

Rotter J. B.: Some problems and misconceptions related to the construct of internal versus external control of reinforcement. *J. Consult Clin Psychol* 43:56-67, 1975.

Sackett D. L., Haynes R. B.: *Compliance with Therapeutic Regimens.* Baltimore, The Johns Hopkins University Press, 1976.

Saltzer E. B.: Locus of control and intention to lose weight. *Health Ed Monogr* 6:118-129, 1978.

Scheiderich S. D.: Registered nurses' knowledge about diabetes mellitus. Paper presented at 4th Annual Nursing Research Forum, U of Illinois, Chicago, February 1980.

Seeley O. F.: Field dependence-independence, internal-external locus of control and implementation of family goals. *Psychol Rep* 38:1216-1218, 1976.

Seeman M., Evans J. W.: Alienation and learning in a hospital setting. *Am Sociol Rev* 27:772-783, 1962.

Sorensen J., Luckmann, J.: *Basic Nursing: A Psychophysiologic Approach.* Philadelphia, W.B. Saunders, 1979.

Squyres W. D. (ed): *Patient Education: An Inquiry into the State of the Art.* New York, Springer Publishing, 1980.

Steffy R. A., Merchenbaum D., Best J. S.: Aversive and cognitive factors in the modification of smokers and nonsmokers. *Behav Res Ther* 8:115-125, 1970.

Straits B., Sechrest L.: Further support of some findings about the characteristics of smokers and nonsmokers. *J Consult Psychol* 27:282, 1963.

Streeter V.: The nurses' responsibility for teaching patients. *Am J. Nurs* 53:818-820, 1953.

Strickland B. R.: Locus of control: Where have we been and where are we going? Paper presented at APA, Montreal, 1973.

Triandis H. C.: *Attitudes and Attitude Change.* New York, J. Wiley and Sons Inc., 1971.

Triandis H. C., Fishbein, M.: Cognitive interaction in person perception. *J Abn Soc Psych* 67:446-453, 1963.

Von Shilling K. C.: The birth of a defective child. *Nurs Forum* 7:424-439, 1968.

Wallston K. A., Maides S., Wallston B. S.: Health-related information-seeking as a function of a health-related locus of control and health value. *J Res Pers* 10:215-222, 1976.

Wallston K. A., Wallston B. S.: Locus of control and health: A review of the literature. *Health Ed Monogr* 6:107-117, 1978.

————: Preface. *Health Ed Monogr* 6:2, 1978.

Wallston K. A., Wallston B. S., DeVellis R.: Development of the Multidimensional health locus of control (mhlc) scales. *Health Ed Monogr* 6:160-170, 1978.

Weiss S. M. (ed): Proceedings of the National Heart and Lung Institute Working Conference on Health Behavior. DHEW Publication No. NIH 76-868 Bethesda, Maryland, Public Health Service, 1975.

Williams A. F.: Factors associated with seat belt use in families. *J Saf Res* 4:133-138, 1972.

————: Personality characteristics associated with preventative dental health practices. *A Am Coll Dent* 39:225-234, 1972.

Author Index

Subject Index

Numbers in italics refer to pages containing tables or diagrams.